DTN

250772

D0502248

WITHDRAWN

Praise from Users of Colette Baron-Reid's Weight-Loss Program

"When you're someone who feels too much, emotional eating can be a real problem. Colette's process gives you tools each step of the way to get back more levels of self-control and self-awareness. With an easy hand she guides you into replacing old habits that aren't working for you anymore with fun new ways of being. The food becomes the way you used to handle stress. Colette rocks!"

—Karen

"This has been a huge lifestyle change for me. I discovered who I am, started loving myself, am now living an authentic life, and lost weight. I'm no longer an active participant in other people's emotions, and I feel 30 pounds lighter in body, mind, and spirit!"

—Cari Friend

"I've tried so many approaches and nothing seemed to 'stick.' This process is different in that it reaches deep, beyond the surface, to the soul level. It gives you a platform where you can be honest and unashamed of feelings that come up when you think about yourself. It has allowed me to find the security, safety, and respect for myself that I've had all along, but that was buried under my actions."

—Patrick Marcoux

"Colette's Weight Release Energetix reached into the core of emotions that cause us to hold on to weight and daily stresses as well. I learned how to respond and to release heavy emotions. My transformation has been amazing from the inside out! I was going into size 14 reluctantly, still trying to squeeze into my size 12 jeans. I am now a size 8!"

—Lisa Springston

"Never before have I felt so empowered to understand myself on such a deep, emotional level! It is this deep understanding that leads to loving control of food choices and self care. I now understand that I can love myself into a thinner, healthier me."

—Kristi Brower

"I have learned that I am much stronger than I have given myself credit for in the past. Situations that have come up over the past few months that normally would have sent me spiraling have not affected me drastically because I now have amazing tools in my back pocket. Yes, weight has been lifted physically from my body, but it is the weight lifted off my spirit that has been so incredibly life changing!"

—Cara Lucia Mansour

Also by Colette Baron-Reid

BOOKS

The Map: Finding the Magic and Meaning in the Story of Your Life

*Messages from Spirit: The Extraordinary Power of
Oracles, Omens, and Signs*

Remembering the Future: The Path to Recovering Intuition

DECKS

The Wisdom of Avalon Oracle Cards: A 52-Card Deck and Guidebook

The Wisdom of the Hidden Realms Oracle Cards

The Enchanted Map Oracle Cards

APPS

The Wisdom of the Hidden Realms

The Wisdom of Avalon

Weight Loss

FOR

People Who Feel Too Much

A 4-STEP, 8-WEEK PLAN
TO FINALLY LOSE THE WEIGHT,
MANAGE EMOTIONAL EATING, AND
FIND YOUR FABULOUS SELF

COLETTE BARON-REID

HARMONY

BOOKS · NEW YORK

Copyright © 2013 by Colette Baron-Reid

All rights reserved.
Published in the United States by Harmony Books, an imprint of
the Crown Publishing Group, a division of Random House, Inc., New York.
www.crownpublishing.com

HARMONY BOOKS is a registered trademark,
and the Circle colophon is a trademark of Random House, Inc.

The IN-VIZION® process is a copyrighted process.
Copyright © 2010 by Colette Baron-Reid. All rights reserved.

IN-VIZION® is a registered U.S. Trademark. Unauthorized use is prohibited.

Weight Release Energetix® is a registered U.S. Trademark.
Unauthorized use is prohibited.

Library of Congress Cataloging-in-Publication Data
is available upon request.

ISBN 978-0-307-98611-5
eISBN 978-0-307-98612-2

Printed in the United States of America

Book design by Jennifer Daddio
Jacket design by Michael Nagin
Jacket photograph: Chris Ryan/Getty Images
Author photograph: Deborah Samuel Photography

10 9 8 7 6 5 4 3 2 1

First Edition

For all those

who feel too much and

have weighed too much,

herein lies hope,

self-love, and freedom

Contents

Part Three: Four Steps to Managing Your Porous Boundaries

Part Four: It's Simple, but It's Not Easy

Author's Note

This book does not claim to dispense any medical advice, nor is it a substitute for medical or psychological treatment. Always consult a physician before beginning any weight-loss plan or taking any supplements, such as those suggested in the book and online program. Results vary from person to person and are not guaranteed.

Names and identifying characteristics have been changed to protect people's privacy.

The Fence

we build this fence around us
high as the sky
made of our beliefs
it
keeps us apart
safe from
what
we do not know
listen with your heart
it has a voice
it
beckons to come closer
see through its cracks
know
the ground beneath it all
shared
a gentle reminder
no need to deny the traveler
nor the journey
loving all these landscapes
sharing every breath
of despair, of love, and hope

—COLETTE BARON-REID

Introduction

What if I said I had a magical formula that would allow you not only to lose the extra weight you're carrying but actually release it effortlessly? What if I told you that after reading this book and working through its four steps, you would make peace with your body and likely never again struggle with your weight?

You'd say, *Yes! I want that NOW!*

Then you'd think I was full of it.

And you'd be right.

Losing weight is not *quite* that easy, but I do know how to help you understand how you got where you are, and how to release the excess weight you can't seem to let go of *and* keep it off. I offer you an approach that I discovered through my own painful struggle and consequent research—an approach that has been unexplored before now. For me, and the hundreds of students who have taken my online class and my Weight Release Coaching Personal Transformation Project, it has been the key to gaining control over distorted and disordered eating and unwanted weight gain.

Weight loss isn't the focus in this program. It's the by-product.

I suspect if you're reading this book that, like me, you've fought your

weight long enough to know there are no quick fixes or enchanted po-
tions available at your local drugstore or through a website. You know
because you've probably tried them all—restrictive diets, pills, affirmations, hypnosis, hormone shots, and even surgery. You may have been
successful at dropping some pounds, but you probably put them all back
on and then some. At times, it probably has seemed that no matter what
you do or don't put in your mouth, your body just wants to swell and
bloat. It's enough to make anyone cuckoo!

You know deep down there's some strong emotional connection that's
made you unable to lose the weight and keep it off, despite your determination and your willingness to devote countless hours and dollars to
learning about and working with weight-loss programs. If you're like me
and the students who have taken my Weight Loss for People Who Feel
Too Much classes, you know there is something different and not right
about why your weight is such an issue. It's more than just what you eat,
more than addiction, more than emotional eating. It's something else
you can't easily put a finger on.

It's about empathy.

Feeling too much is all about the ability to sense the world beyond
your own personal boundaries, and becoming overwhelmed not just by
your own feelings—we all know about that—but also by feelings that
don't belong to you, that are "out there" in the environment. Although
that ability to connect can be a great asset, it can also make you fat.

Try this quiz and see if you are a person who feels too much. Is your
empathy overload affecting your weight?

• THE EMPATHY AND EATING QUIZ •

For each question, circle Y for yes or N for no.

1. You feel overwhelmed by your emotions around certain people,
    and don't always know if your emotions belong to you. Y/N

2. You feel disconnected and disoriented by strong emotions during
    family encounters, and you turn to food to calm down. Y/N

3. You turn to food as comfort or reward, and to calm yourself or to escape your feelings, especially from 4:00 P.M. on. Y/N

4. When you feel emotionally unsafe, food is temporarily calming and makes you feel grounded and secure, if only for a few seconds. Y/N

5. There are times when, rather than face a social opportunity, you stay home and eat comfort foods that may be a combination of sugar, flour, and dairy or are processed foods such as chips, cookies, etc. Y/N

6. Sometimes, you can't stop eating these comfort foods, and you mentally bargain with yourself that you will start again on Monday (or tomorrow). Y/N

7. During stressful times, you can gain weight without eating extra food. Y/N

8. In your experience, fear and excess food go together. Y/N

9. You gain weight as soon as you think about dieting. Y/N

10. You feel afraid that you won't ever get your eating under control. Y/N

11. You feel powerless when you're in an emotional eating phase and powerful when you think you've got it handled. Y/N

12. Your love/sex life has suffered because of your relationship to food. Y/N

If you answered yes to three or more questions, your empathy is probably interfering with your ability to lose weight and keep it off.

The latest research into weight loss has taught us that metabolism, or the "set point" for your weight, is influenced by many factors. How many calories you take in and expend through exercise and activity is only part of the picture. For instance, you've probably noticed that it's much harder to lose weight when you're under emotional, psychological stress. You may even know the physical reason for that (if you don't, I promise you'll know after reading this book!).

The truth is that your excess weight may have very little to do with food! In recent years, scientists such as Bruce Lipton, Ph.D., and Candace Pert, Ph.D., have alerted us to the actual physiological changes that occur in our cells and our bodies as a result of our thoughts and emotions.

It makes sense that our fat can start with fear, anger, or an unwillingness to let go of emotions and thoughts that affect us on a physiological level. People who are exquisitely sensitive, who feel more deeply and experience other people's emotions as their own, often have quite a struggle losing weight and keeping it off. Could it be that the wonderful quality of empathy, which allows them to truly feel other people's pain and express compassion, is a major factor in their weight problems?

Weight Loss for People Who Feel Too Much is not a typical weight-loss book. I'm not offering you a mechanistic formula to achieve success. Instead, I'm going to help you discover the hidden causes for weight gain and obesity so that you can address them at last. I know what you're thinking: "Yeah yeah, sounds good. But what about the cookies? *Do I get to eat the cookies?*" Well . . . maybe. Only if they are not trigger foods for you that set off emotional drama, and you eat them consciously. Even then, they may have to be sugar- and gluten-free, given your unique situation. And you can only have a few, served on a plate. Eating has to have a beginning, a middle, and an end, and it can't be used as a distraction or entertainment. Otherwise, for people who feel too much, eating becomes a detour away from emotional stress that needs to be managed.

I'm not going to be the captain of the food police, but I'm also not going to let you give up on reaching a healthy BMI (body mass index). You *can* achieve that. I'll talk to you frankly about food and your eating habits, but not until later in the book. First, you have to start managing your porous boundaries: you are taking in stimulation and agitation from outside of you and absorbing the emotions of others until you're on empathy overload—and as a result, you are gaining weight. You are actually taking on the "weight of the world." And could it also be possible that you're solidifying it in your body by your thoughts of self-reproach and anger for gaining weight? Your own feelings about the weight you've gained from absorbing the feelings of others are like adding glue to it all to ensure those extra pounds surely will stay put! Well, I'm here to explain how you can avoid that complicated mess and manage your boundaries so that you don't feel overwhelmed and run to the cookie jar.

I know from experience how easy it is to obsess about food and exercise as a way of avoiding the more difficult work of facing your painful emotions, so I'm asking you to be patient. I am going to show you how to sort out those feelings, how to find out which are your feelings and which are from outside of yourself. I'm also going to show you how to release the feelings so you can release the weight. It's the *feelings* that keep you fat.

So we'll get to the food later—but first, you need to understand the weight you carry (Part I of the book) and commit to a simple plan for working this program (Part II). Then you'll be ready to begin taking the four steps of this program, which are explained in Part III. Each step will require your intense attention for an entire week, and you'll follow that with a week of processing what you've learned and experienced emotionally:

Step One. Speak your truth. Acknowledge your struggle with weight and the fact that what you've done in the past never worked for very long. This step asks you to get really honest with yourself as you explore your personal story. Why? Because you need to see clearly for yourself how your story with food, weight, feelings, and porous boundaries has affected you. Once you get out of denial, the lightbulb will go on. You will see how your emotional sensitivity to your environment affects you. You'll come to recognize your behavioral, thinking, and feeling patterns and you'll find that you will never be able to eat mindlessly, nor engage in negative self-talk, and remain at a healthy weight for you. That's okay, because you're going to learn how to eat mindfully and process your emotions rather than avoid them. You're also going to learn how to recognize when your porous boundaries are wide open and taking in all the dreck that's out there.

Step Two. Own your truth. It's one thing to acknowledge intellectually what you've been denying for a long time. It's another thing to emotionally accept it. This step often causes the most resistance, but I'm here to help you break through it. This is where you will start seeing the effects of using specific techniques for setting and maintaining healthy boundaries for yourself. I'll talk about the importance of bringing joy back into your life, and feeling gratitude for your body. You'll learn why relying on a higher power, a force larger than yourself that can support you and nurture in a way that food can't, can be extremely helpful. In fact, recognizing a greater infinite intelligence, or Spiritual Source, is essential for success in this program. I'll provide liberating exercises for feeling a sense of connection to this loving higher power, for appreciating your body's health and stamina, and for remembering that you are not alone on your journey. Help can be immediate once you make a shift in perception, set your intention, and employ your imagination to release the weight you're holding.

Step Three. Reclaim your power to choose. The only way to put an end to the old, mindless eating habits is to develop self-awareness and self-compassion. When you beat yourself up for overeating, you backslide, then feel guilty and ashamed, then give up on yourself. When you love yourself enough to stop, forgive yourself, explore what happened, and have faith in your ability to get it right the next time, you make progress. The goal is progress, not perfection. Self-love is the key to reclaiming your power to make conscious choices in the moment, to follow through on your commitment to the simple plan for eating right and managing your porous boundaries.

Step Four. Reconnect without losing yourself. When you live in fear and judge yourself harshly, it dims your light: you feel depressed, weighed down, and unmotivated. In this very important step, you're going to find the courage to stop making yourself small and hiding your brilliance and beauty. You'll reconnect with your body, mind, and spirit, as well as with other people. You'll learn how to create healthy boundaries and how to balance the desire to isolate with the desire to have emotional connections, so that you're no longer avoiding people or enmeshing with them.

Commit to the four steps for eight weeks. The week devoted to doing the exercises, including journal writing, may be intense for you emotionally. That's why it's important to spend that second week of the step continuing the basic exercises and processing what you have learned and felt. As you'll discover, we people who feel too much take in so much information and emotion on a daily basis that we become easily overwhelmed and shut down. Then we head straight for the pantry and the bag of chips.

Don't underestimate the importance of that second, less demanding week. If you find the work harder than expected and need more time before going on to each consecutive step, then go ahead and take a little longer to work the step or process the information. However, you'll need to become aware of your detours, from procrastination and perfectionism to caretaking and disordered eating, and pull yourself back onto the main road!

In Part IV of this book, I turn to the topic of food and give you guidance on how to eat nutritious foods that are cruelty-free and grown sustainably. You'll get specific advice on what to eat to support your well-being. Again, please don't skip ahead and detour away from the main work in the four steps of the Weight Loss for People Who Feel Too Much program.

In the last chapter of the book, I guide you through exceptionally challenging times in your personal life that can trigger disordered eating and weight gain. I deliberately scheduled the very first telecourse of the Weight Loss for People Who Feel Too Much program to take place during the holidays because I know how hard it is to deal with festive tables loaded with treats, emotional scenes involving troubled family dynamics, and the constant exhortation to "celebrate the season"—meaning, "throw your rules about food and exercise out the window." You can have fun without using food to cope, and you don't have to isolate yourself to turn down the volume on your emotions.

Although this will be a very personal journey for you, and you'll do a lot of self-discovery and self-growth, by working with the Weight Loss for People Who Feel Too Much program, you'll be making it easier to connect with a world that's in transformation. All of us are undergoing an extraordinary evolution in the human experience, and that's contributing to the challenge of managing your porous boundaries, your emotions, your mental stimulation, and your weight. I'll give you some solid advice on staying grounded and centered as we all face the rapid changes that are happening globally.

You'll no longer have to reach for the chocolate to bring you back into your body and your own psyche. Now you'll have the tools you need to be fully present in times of uncertainty and emotional agitation without feeling the need to run and hide or put up a fight and battle the world, yourself, or your weight. Get ready to discover how to release the extra pounds, and the emotional burdens you may have carried inside you your whole life, and free yourself to have a new, healthy relationship with your body, your weight, and food.

PART ONE

Understanding the Weight You Carry

Feeling Too Much:
The Hidden Thread

I don't remember what was causing the tension to swirl through our house like the winds of autumn, sending emotional debris spinning through the air with such intensity that it seemed to smack up against me. What I do remember was what I felt like: confused and unsafe, as if the stories I could sense on the outside somehow got inside of me. I was helplessly floating in the chaos that surrounded and penetrated me. I was only four years old, but I remember the experience vividly.

I had to have relief. *Make it stop!* I had to close myself off, ground myself in my body, in Colette.

I knew just what to do. I picked up a cooking spoon that had sticky raw cake dough on it, and as soon as I put it in my mouth, I felt calm. Now, that feeling didn't last, but it was very powerful. I had already discovered the connection between food and self-soothing. The fear melted away as the gooey, sweet mess on that spoon dissolved in my mouth and slid down my throat. I was "home," in a safe place where that icky feeling of something being very wrong couldn't get inside me again. That sense of physicality as the cake dough entered my body gave me a sense of substance. It made me feel whole, and secure.

It would be years before I understood this experience or its signifi-cance, but when I finally did, everything changed. I realized that the missing piece in the puzzle of my baffling relationship to food, eating, and weight was *empathy*. I was a person who felt too much, and I was using food to detour away from the awful feeling of not knowing where I ended and others began.

Food sealed my porous boundaries where other people's energy in-vaded me, and it allowed me to feel present in myself. I needed that quiet and calm, but I had to find a better way to achieve it. This revelation ended an exhausting war with food and my weight and began a new chapter for me. While I'm not a size 2, and I can't claim to have the figure of a 20-year-old high-fashion model, most of the time I'm at peace with my body and myself. That alone is an incredible feat, given how much I have struggled with all of this over the years.

It was this missing piece of feeling too much that allowed me to stop beating myself up (which, as it turns out, is counterproductive when try-ing to lose weight, as you'll learn later in this book). Once I did that, I started to better understand the many influences on those formerly dys-functional relationships between myself, food, and my body. I was able to address those influences, too—but it all began with understanding why I was feeling too much and why fear and frustration were making me fat.

POROUS BOUNDARIES

A person who feels too much often senses the need to eat because her experience of the world is too much for her. It's not that she simply loves the taste, texture, smell, and sight of food, which provides a sensory ex-perience. It's not that she's experiencing hunger pangs, or even that she's addicted to food, although that may be. Diets don't work for her because they don't address her powerful need to feel grounded in herself, sepa-rated from the confusing, distressing emotional turbulence around her. Food serves that purpose.

The stress of remaining in the moment, without knowing what you are sensing and how to be separate from it, is deeply discombobulating for someone who feels too much. The pain and discomfort are intolerable, and you will do anything to escape.

If you're highly sensitive and empathetic, that has a profound influence on your weight, as well as your thought processes and your moods, which affect your eating habits and your relationships with others. I'm sure you know all about emotional eating, but you've probably never considered what empathetic eating is. There is a subtle yet profound difference between the two. An example of emotional eating would be feeling so uncomfortable after a conflict with a coworker that you reach for the stash of mini candy bars you keep in your desk drawer to calm your anger and embarrassment.

However, let's say that it's not you who was in conflict with someone at work but two people in another department. You walk into the meeting room where they just had a heated argument and you feel the tension in the air. You're unsettled and uncomfortable and have no clue why. As other coworkers file into the meeting room, you have a compelling urge to sneak back to your office and grab some candy bars. You start feeling defensive and on alert, and you can't understand why. All you know is that you want those mini chocolates right now. That's empathetic eating.

Emotional eating and empathetic eating often occur at the same time. Let's say you're about to leave for work and you're feeling particularly vulnerable because you woke up, weighed yourself, and were embarrassed and ashamed by the number on the scale. You drive to work and feel frustrated, anxious, and angry that other cars aren't allowing you to merge. Then you walk into the meeting room where tension hangs in the air and you suddenly realize there's a ball of confusing emotions rolling around inside you and you have no idea how to sort it out. Visions of doughnuts dance in your head. Your emotions are difficult enough to deal with, but now you've taken on the emotions of others and added them to the mix. You've done this because you're highly sensitive and empathetic, and other people's emotions flood into you through your porous boundaries.

You probably don't realize when you're taking on someone else's emotions that you're experiencing feelings that aren't yours. Thoughts don't enter your mind when you're deeply upset and feeling ungrounded. You just feel discombobulated, or upset. You can't put your finger on what you're really feeling. You don't say, "Hey there, self. Bob's anger has entered you and you're tuned in to him!" All you know is that you have to have that salty, sugary, fatty treat *now*.

I know what this is like because I have felt this way with disturbing regularity: filled with confusing emotions that were upsetting me. I didn't recognize that many of those feelings weren't even mine. Why did it take me so long to figure this out? Why don't diet books or courses teach us about how taking on other people's "stuff" affects us? In our culture, we don't talk much about empathy, so when you're sitting there feeling guilty for downing a huge portion of junk food, you're not likely to think about this whole "empathy" and "sensitivity" thing. But ah, if you did, what you would learn!

WHAT IT'S LIKE TO BE DEEPLY EMPATHETIC

Empathy is much underrated. From childhood, we learn that brute strength, toughness, and smarts are what we need to succeed and be happy in life. We rarely celebrate sensitivity, or the beauty of caring deeply. Too often, sensitivity is seen as a weakness, something to be ashamed of (and more so for men than for women, which is why sensitive men have it especially rough).

But being empathetic—feeling others' emotions as your own—can give you a deeper understanding of others and greater compassion. If you're highly sensitive and empathetic, your friends probably would say you're the one person they can always count on to know they're sad when they're pretending everything is okay. You can probably sense feelings others don't pick up on. That sensitivity enables you to "read" situations very well and respond accordingly. Your actions and decisions take into account the hidden reality of people's emotions. You might find that people seem instinctively drawn to you, and random strangers may even tell you their troubles. I have a friend who is hopeless at directions, but whenever she's in New York City, strangers push their way through crowds to ask her to point them to Broadway. She just gives off an approachable and kind energy—and then she has to admit that she has no idea whether she and the stranger are facing north, south, east, or west.

Your intuitiveness and sensitivity may make you an excellent healer, teacher, and counselor. You may play that role in your relationships—the "unpaid psychiatrist" of all your friends or the harmony establisher in your family. Or, you may actually work in the helping professions as a therapist, nurse, doctor, social worker, acupuncturist, executive assistant, or in human resources, and so on, or perhaps you work in a creative, artistic field. You probably see other people in shades of gray rather than black or white, and you don't overidentify with one separate group. Ultimately, feeling "too much" can be quite an asset, personally and professionally. Take a minute to feel how wonderful that is.

And when you feel more intensely than others do, you can truly revel in shared experiences, like concerts, picnics, or spiritual gatherings. You don't just have fun on these occasions. You feel sheer joy filling every pore in your body, and you soak in the pleasure of everyone around you. Heaven!

But let's face it, there's a down side, too. If you feel too much, even happy experiences can quickly make you feel overstimulated or hyper, which can trigger anxiety because that sense of excitement seems out of your control. You start feeling ungrounded and anxious, and begin looking for a sanctuary from all the hoopla. You have to develop coping mechanisms. It's all too much.

You may even have begun early in life sensing the world too much as unsafe so you spend most of your life isolated from others. I know some empathetic people who completely numb out and shut down, unable to feel anything at all because it's too scary. To heck with feelings—you might have even developed a very strong personality to ensure that you can control who connects with you and who doesn't. And guess who needs to always be in control of that dial, more than likely on the "Don't come near me unless I say how, when, and exactly for how long" setting? There's a whole spectrum of coping mechanisms that people who feel too much engage in to avoid the onslaught of feelings picked up like lint floating through the emotional environment. You may cope by having your "radar" constantly on Alert to ensure that the vibes you pick up are turned right down or off, even if they are wonderful and meant to be comforting. Don't hug me, don't touch me, don't stand so close to me! You're not having any of that!

On top of that, the vibes you're feeling aren't always pleasant, anyway. People's anger easily rattles you, even when it's just a shouting match on a reality TV show. When someone is callous or insensitive, you feel uneasy. This is true even if the person's behavior isn't directed at you but, rather, at someone else. If you hear about people or animals suffering, you just can't bear it. Grief or anger settles over you like a dark, heavy blanket and it dampens your mood for hours, even days.

Is it possible that loving and caring for others, being generous and openhearted, can make you fat? Consider: why are so many nurses overweight? As they take care of the sick, who is taking care of them? How are they processing what they see, experience, and feel all day long as they work their high-stress jobs? Although obesity rates are rising in all communities, in his book *Microtrends*, Mark Penn points out that African-American women are three times as likely as any other subgroup of Americans to be overweight. The women most likely to be morbidly obese are the caregivers in their communities—the full-time grandmothers, the nurses and nurses' aides, the church volunteers, and the teachers. It can't be just about the food they are eating. Could it be that these women are taking on the weight of their overburdened communities?

What if, instead of beating yourself up for being overweight, you appreciated your kindness, sensitivity, compassion, and generosity? What if you made a commitment to show yourself and your body the love you show to others? What if you came out of isolation and allowed yourself to *feel*? What if you stepped back from your emotions and your persistent inner critic, and instead told yourself, *You are a treasure. I am so honored to know you, to actually be you.*

Try it.

This is what you *need to start doing*. It may be uncomfortable at first, but with practice, you are going to become kinder to yourself. That alone will be a strong foundation for bringing your body back to its optimum health and weight. Love thyself. Love thy body. You will be amazed at how much power you have to change what you wish to change when you start with *love*.

So how did you get here? How did your empathy, and the other factors in your complex relationships with your body and your food, affect you?

A LIFE'S TAPESTRY: FINDING PATTERNS
IN THE FABRIC OF YOUR REALITY

What if you could look at your life as if it were a giant tapestry, woven with brightly colored threads that tell the story of you? The fabric of your reality would be so easy to understand! Imagine that the threads going across represent your life experiences and the conditions of your life—your family, friends, opportunities. The way you respond to those conditions, with or without awareness, determines the vertical threads. Wouldn't it be great to have such a tangible depiction of your life experiences? Then, it would be so easy to understand how you got from A to B in your story. You would be able to see all the repetitive patterns that have marked your life and could recognize their origins. *Here is where this one begins, and here is where that one begins. Look there! That one stopped repeating. That pattern in the tapestry only happened once and never again.*

Your issues with food and your body would show up in one or two obvious colors, which would make it easy to see the conditions that caused the pattern to repeat—and keep repeating. Then you would have a thread representing your feelings. It would be so easy to recognize how your emotions and your relationships to food and your body come together. This pattern might run continuously through the whole tapestry. The patterns would change according to your choices or would repeat when you didn't, wouldn't, or maybe couldn't make a choice that might alter them. You could discover the conditions that trigger your issues by looking at the way the threads that represent them cause the pattern to shift. From that outside perspective, you could see what you couldn't when you were *inside* the tapestry, aware of your experiences and emotions but unaware of the patterns they were weaving.

Looking at your life as a tapestry, you'd find that all the troublesome issues you've faced would finally make sense, because you could follow the threads woven into the pattern and find the place where the pattern changed into something new. *Here's where I lost weight; here's where I started to gain it again; here's where I kept hating my body, which made me get even fatter; here's where I tried to control things. Here are the same conditions that repeated earlier! Here is where I dieted and gained weight; here's where I ate well but couldn't lose the weight. Right here is where the threads got all twisted and balled up and left a hole.*

"What's this?" you ask. "Did some crazy phantom weaver wreck my tapestry? How did I not notice this?"

Somehow, another colored thread got in there and changed the pattern. When you look closer, you can separate that thread, finding its beginning and tracing how it parallels all the other threads in the pattern. Why didn't you or anyone else notice this rogue thread? It's always there when the pattern gets twisted or a hole appears. This is the thread that represents empathy: the ability to sense the bonds between all living things and, especially, the emotional energies of others. As you peer closely at this thread, you ponder why it wrecks the pattern or leaves a hole in the tapestry.

Wouldn't it be great if it were that easy to discover the roots of our problems and behavior patterns? Find the thread, untangle it, fill the hole. Snip, snip—tapestry repaired. We'd have instant food control, wouldn't hate our bodies any longer, wouldn't isolate ourselves or be too sensitive to the moods of the universe and its breathing population. If understanding how weight issues and tendencies to feel overwhelmed by the world were as easy as following the threads in a tapestry, you wouldn't need this book.

But if you identify with my story and with others in these pages, you will start to see how the unique and confusing strands in the tapestry of your reality form a pattern. Then you'll get the relief, understanding, and information you need to stop the struggle to release the excess weight sticking to you like a puffy coat. You'll learn to love and accept yourself, and to find ways to manage your emotions, especially the emotions outside of you that have gotten all mixed up with your own. So, bear with me while I show you the individual strands that make up the most perplexing and challenging patterns that lead to the dysfunctional relationship many of us have to food, feelings, and fat.

I know I am not alone in this because, as an intuitive counselor, coach, and life strategist for the past twenty-three years, I have met thousands of people who are just like me. Maybe you are one of them, too? We are people who have three things in common that up until now have not been correlated:

1. *We have little or no control over our weight.* Weight can fluctuate without changing what we eat, and dieting does not work (and we've tried everything).
2. *We feel too much!* It's hard for us to be around people because the feelings we experience are not always our own, but in fact may be ones we've picked up from others. We get cuckoo going through a crowd because we feel bombarded by their emotions. This makes us feel mixed up, and by the end of the day, we're overwhelmed by the multitude of feelings we've taken on.
3. *We generally have a disordered relationship with food and our bodies, although we've had periods of relief from this that may or may not have resulted in weight loss.* Nutritional nourishment isn't the number one reason why we eat. We may even have stretches when eating healthfully is not an issue and we feel on top of the world, but then it all goes down the toilet.

Have I gotten your attention? Could you belong to the People Who Feel Too Much Club?

I know I do. And I have found a way to manage the feeling of being overwhelmed that comes with that membership package. I can help you release the excess weight you're carrying, whether it be on your thighs or butt, or weighing down your mind.

Before we continue, I want to ask you not to compare your story to mine, or the others in this book. Rather, see what you can identify with.

It's the essence of the story that counts, not the details. Also, remember that these threads are sometimes so tightly woven that it takes a while to pull them apart, so be patient with yourself.

MY STORY: FOOD, FEELINGS, AND EMPATHY

Looking back over my life, it's easy for me to see how I have always had a deeply passionate and wildly dysfunctional relationship with food. I am, in fact, a flag-flying, self-confessed foodie! I love food! Food has been my friend, my medicine, and my answer to boredom, rejection, and fear of rejection. It has been a celebration of happiness and an antidote to sadness. Until I learned what I share with you in this book, food gave me a reason to avoid and procrastinate, and to escape anything that I could imagine needing escape from—responsibility, accountability, sex, and power—although I couldn't see it at the time. I never gave eating much real thought. Eating was my go-to instinct whenever I craved safety. The fact that food had something also to do with nutrition interested me only when I was trying to control my weight. Food was a festivity, an encounter, a senses-filled experience! Food was a living companion with a personality.

I even argued with it!

Why are you doing this to me?

Ooo! Yummy! I love you so much!!!

Then right, afterward:

I hate you! Blechh! You're going in the garbage!

Wait—don't go. I need you now. I can start again, and never taste you for the rest of my life, on Monday!

You are disgusting and you make me sick!

If I eat you standing up, you won't hurt me, right? Just a little?

I don't think it's normal to have such heated discussions with a chocolate cookie.

At age three, whenever I cried, the only thing that would shut me up was to give me a crust of bread or a cookie to suck on. Then I would happily gurgle away in the corner. I also didn't like to be hugged. I would push everyone away, but if someone did manage to grab me for longer than a few moments, I would immediately beg for a sweet or anything else that I could put in my mouth that was edible—including dog biscuits, much to the chagrin of our golden retriever. Take note of this, as I will discuss this very important parallel thread of sensitivity later; that was an early sign that I was a person who feels too much. (Hint: I needed to eat something after I had contact with another person's energy. *That lady hugged me and squeezed my cheeks! Help! I'm being invaded!*)

Part of my complex emotional relationship with food was based on my relationship with my mother. She hid from me a secret past of being a Holocaust survivor, and her subsequent fears of being unsafe and starving; in part, I continuously intruded on her psychic space (which I wrote about at length in my first two books). There was intense connection and much love between us, although it seems to me that the love was almost always expressed through food. For me, "mother" was associated with food and nurturing—and there was confusion about where I ended and she began.

For many people who feel too much, food has become a substitute for the missing maternal force, whether it's because they grew up without a mother, Mom had her own issues and couldn't be nurturing, or she couldn't keep her baby safe from abuse and harm, for all that she tried.

Like many people who feel too much, my relationship with food changed at adolescence, a time when we assert our own, individual identity and discover our autonomy and sexuality. Freak me out! I chafed at my parents' control over me and the lack of personal privacy and boundaries in my home. I began to connect with the frightening truth of my sexuality, and I sensed the "otherness" of my own self and my body. To regain control, a few weeks after I started menstruating, I began bingeing and purging. Then I discovered diet pills and spent years trying every diet or intervention I could find. Even so, my feeling of not knowing where I ended and others began continued to haunt me.

As I moved toward adulthood, I couldn't tell if I was feeling my feelings, if I was reacting to sensing others' feelings, or what was going on. My hunger was to feel safe inside my skin and to plug those holes I couldn't see. I knew they were there, though. People who feel too much always know their boundaries are porous; they just don't know how to say it, how to manage it, or what it really means to them.

I hope by now you're beginning to identify some things we have in common. Although my story is extreme—you may not have been obsessed with food, addicted, bulimic, or anorexic—the pattern of distorted eating, emotional agitation, and confusion about boundaries is the same for all people who feel too much. The patterns begin long before they reveal themselves as a problem.

By age 27, I was a full-blown drug addict and alcoholic, on top of having many issues with food. My life wasn't working, there was no escape, and by the grace of Spirit, I hit bottom. On January 2, 1986, I woke up clean and sober, and have been so a day at a time ever since. Though I continued to struggle with food, weight, and empathy overload, I began to sort out all my addictions and issues. I learned a lot about controlling my weight and eating when I was in Overeaters Anonymous, which I joined after I stopped drinking and I began to gain weight. There, I heard from many people who shared the same experiences I'd had—weight gain that couldn't be explained by a simple equation of calories in, calories out. We all knew and understood that out-of-control emotions often led us to overeat, or to eat mindlessly. For me, that mysterious-weight-gain piece just hung out there, a cipher that I hoped would explain itself someday. Meanwhile, the numbers on my scale went up and down, which challenged my self-esteem. I hated not being able to control my weight, and I wore my shame and frustration in every extra pound.

Then, as I became more confident in my sobriety and worked through some of the more painful issues, thereby developing a stronger sense of self-worth and self-esteem, I found that with very little effort on my part, the pounds just started coming off. *Wow, what was that about? Who cares? Something's working! I'm getting thinner! Woo hoo!* I was lead singer and songwriter in an all-girl group called Isis, and I was loving my life. Singing was medicine. The more I sang, the more grounded I felt. I was finally doing what made me happy and inspired me. One of my musician friends was a student of Tibetan Buddhism, and he seemed always "chill" and relaxed; since I was definitely *not* that, I joined a meditation group as part of my new healthy lifestyle.

A health food store near my home sold Himalayan salts for the bath, and in conversation with the owner one day, I told him I was on a clean-living path. He suggested using the baths as a detox and calmative, and I started to meditate while taking salt baths before bed as the final part of my daily routine. I ate well, without too many restrictions (I avoided white sugar and flour, but that's about it—although that's a key to my maintaining a healthy weight today, too). I exercised moderately, walking for about an hour a day. Each day, I had a plan. As suggested in twelve-step programs, I turned my will and my life and my food and my body over to a higher power. I'd created this structure to ensure my mental, spiritual, and physical wellness, and I found it made me feel liberated regardless of the outer conditions of my life that were mired in stress.

My father had lost all the family's money in a bad business venture a few years before this, and both my parents became ill from the stress. My father developed rapid-onslaught Alzheimer's disease and then died of a stroke. Somehow I stayed sober and clean and numb, without too big a detour into foodville. It appeared I could handle everything that life threw at me—no problem. Then, a year later, everything changed.

I was 138 pounds the day my mom was diagnosed with cancer. By her funeral four months later, I weighed 219 pounds. I did not eat enough calories to have gained 80 pounds in less than four months! This bizarre weight gain when my mom died was the first, most obvious sign that there was some mysterious thread affecting my life tapestry that I needed to discern and understand. The fact that feelings alone could make me fat was unthinkable, unscientific, and impossible—yet I couldn't deny what had just happened. I stayed very heavy for another couple of years, ignoring many of my good habits other than not picking up a drink or drug. Nothing miraculous occurred the day I surrendered, but I guess you might say I just got sick and tired of being sick and tired; and so I began to embark on a new journey of self-acceptance, working with a therapist, meditating again, and being honest with myself about my detours.

Things improved again, I met a man, and I married him, in spite of the warnings from friends (and his mother, now a dear friend). Of course, the weight started climbing back on, slowly but surely like a creeping vine. The marriage was steeped in sarcasm and lack of mutual respect, and food yet again became my solace. I relentlessly dieted, to no avail. One day, I finally just stopped fighting and accepted that I had no power to change anything. I was defeated, and I surrendered to the real truth of what was happening to me and to my strained relationship with my husband.

To be true to myself, and to stop the cycle of suffering, I walked out of that marriage. I looked at myself as I was, and I figured that if this was it, I would learn to love and forgive myself, and treat myself the way I needed to be treated. No one else would be able to do that for me. I took out a photograph of me when I was a little girl, and I propped it up by my bedside and promised that little girl that I would love and protect her.

I simplified my life, I began meditating again, and I limited sugar and flour in my food. There was no diet; I just went back to what I knew worked from my core, and not because I had a too detailed plan. I started to use the gorgeous soaker tub in my new apartment. Salt baths were my nightly treat! The more I loved myself just as I was, the faster things changed. I began exercising moderately again—a little yoga, dancing, walking, and doing some light weight training. The pounds began to drop off as if by magic.

I began to notice the pattern and the relationships between feeling too much of the environment I was exposed to, the stress due to my weight fluctuations, my eating patterns, and my feeling of being emotionally overwhelmed. The detours began to become more and more obvious. Could it be that I finally found that rogue thread in the fabric that had been hidden from me until now?

WEIGHT AND LIFE STAGES

Being overwhelmed by feelings has been a common experience for me ever since I was a small child, and this has never changed fundamentally. It has been acutely noticeable in cycles, depending on what was happening in my life. Your story may have similar threads. We all go through stages and changes, and those of us who feel too much can be profoundly affected by a big emotional shift. Teenagers on the whole are hormonal messes, which makes it difficult to perform the job of adolescence: to find one's identity. When you don't know where you end and others begin, that separation is even more unsettling. Motherhood and pregnancy can bring up issues of separateness and togetherness, of loving your child without losing yourself, of having to trust that you can become a good mother. One of my friends was excited to see that the 37 pounds she gained during pregnancy dropped off in a week after she gave birth, and credited the weight loss to breastfeeding. Her delight was short-lived, as all the weight crept back in a few weeks, even though she went back to her pre-pregnancy eating habits. "My baby wasn't nursing properly; I knew there was something wrong with him, and people were doubting my instincts. My mom had gone back home, and now the weight of being a mom was fully on me—and apparently, on my butt, belly, and thighs as well!"

Midlife brings all of us new emotional stressors as we assess what we've done or didn't do up to this point in our lives, and we begin to recognize that the consequences of our choices over the years weren't necessarily what we expected. Caretaking for children, our elders, or close friends who unexpectedly become ill stir up more emotions. One of the participants in my online class told me that she had always been incredibly vigilant with her weight, controlling herself well, being mindful of never going past a size 6. She was so proud of herself. She admitted the control was always on her mind, and she spent hours sometimes deciding she would not have the evil piece of cake. Then her sister got cancer and she became her caretaker. She felt very conflicted about it because she and her sister had not gotten along, although she loved her dearly and felt obliged to help. She was angry that she was inconvenienced, guilty because she felt angry, and terrified of losing her sister. She began eating more because, well, it made her feel better. She added an extra piece of this, a helping of that, choosing fast foods on the way to the hospital, adding wine when she got home. She came to my class a year later, a size 16, exhausted and filled with fear. Her sister recovered, but she found herself the one needing help.

Menopause, and becoming an "elder of the tribe," as well as losing our parents, brings to the surface unresolved issues and, with them, fears of abandonment. You feel that as an elder, you are responsible for all the problems in society that need fixing. You're supposed to clean up the mess and offer wisdom. This is the time you should be feeling more secure, yet that feeling can elude you, especially if you may have seen the shifts in the economy eat away at your retirement security. You can't help watching the news, and as you fill yourself with information you can barely process, and fears course through your body, your boundaries become weaker and *kaboom!* You're in Chubbyville.

If you look at your life tapestry and focus on increments of time, you discover how empathy has affected you as you began to be aware of your surroundings, you piled the emotions of others on top of your own feelings, and as a consequence, you isolated yourself or found other detours to avoid the intensity of what you were experiencing. Look closely, and you also begin to see the patterns that connect your emotional issues and your unique relationships to food and weight.

ARE WE ALL GETTING MORE EMPATHIC?

You and I are not alone in feeling too much and in struggling with the discomfort of being overly sensitive and empathetic. Elaine Aron, author of *The Highly Sensitive Person,* estimates the number of highly sensitive people to be around 20 percent of the population. I believe the number may have grown larger since she did her research because, as Jeremy Rifkin, expert in economics and international affairs, explained in his book *The Empathic Civilization,* we're experiencing a far greater and more intense sense of connection to other people at this stage of human evolution. Globally, 845 million (that's 1 in 8) people are on Facebook, and software and applications are allowing them to connect Facebook to other social media on a variety of telecommunications devices at the touch of a button. The Arab Spring came about because of a passionate message and cry that spread virally, person to person, through Twitter and on smartphones. Technology communications are changing the human experience rapidly. Are we really up for this?

How are you supposed to feel when we're in a world that's more connected than ever? How do you constantly confront information you need to process not just intellectually but emotionally? You can be standing in line for coffee, checking a social media site or your e-mail on your smartphone, and find out that a former schoolmate or your cousin's husband just got diagnosed with cancer. Or, you're home, bored, and you pick up the television remote and start clicking your way to your favorite channel, then suddenly see graphic crime photos of a murder victim. Some people aren't emotionally affected by these experiences, but you sure are.

Around the world, unemployment rates are high and people are worried about finances more than ever before. Our institutions are dysfunctional, we have no idea how to fix them or where we're headed, and everyone seems to be arguing and hurling insults at each other. Every day there are stories to trigger you, from the implication of nuclear war to the looming threat of currency devaluation, recession, and more. Then, when you decide you can't take the serious news anymore and you reach for a gossip magazine at the grocery store, you see stories and photos of movie stars far thinner than you are being ridiculed for being fat!

How does it feel to pick up on all that every day? Bombarded by stories about financial threats, or being too fat, do you start thinking, "OMG, I need to go on a diet!" or "Gee, today would be a good day for a martini—with a giant bowl of bar snacks"? Some people aren't easily tempted by racks of chips and sugary sodas, which seem to be within reach wherever we go. Some people aren't experiencing information overload, and they don't feel overwhelmed by the emotional turbulence. Maybe they compartmentalize their emotions better than we people who feel too much, or they easily talk themselves out of worrying about people and situations they can't influence.

It's likely that these people just are not wired, as we are, for extreme empathy. They have "thicker" boundaries. But if you're more sensitive, more empathetic, you're likely to struggle with your weight and with disordered eating. You are taking on the weight of the world, figuratively and literally.

How does this work, exactly? How does fear become fat, and how does frustration end up on your belly and thighs? Let's look next at the way our weight is influenced by the energy field we share with each other, and the research that shows its physical effects on us.

KEEP IN MIND . . .

- We're able to take on others' emotional energy and feel what they feel. This experience is called *empathy,* and people who feel too much are more empathetic than most.
- Humans are becoming more empathetic because we're all more connected than we have been in the past.
- The discomfort of empathy overload causes people who feel too much to shut down and withdraw from social interactions, and to detour into behaviors such as overindulging in food. We turn to food to feel grounded in our own physicality, separate from the confusing jumble of emotions we're experiencing. Our eating becomes disordered as a result.
- Empathy overload can also cause weight gain that seems to defy logic.
- At very stressful times in our lives, we are more likely to be overwhelmed by our emotions and respond with disordered eating.
- To release the weight of the world we are carrying emotionally, energetically, and physically, we must develop the ability to close up our porous boundaries and manage our empathy. Then it will be easier to address any disordered eating.
- To start this process of learning to manage our porous boundaries, we need to look back at the threads in the tapestry of our lives and see how feelings, foods, and our relationship to our bodies are intertwined. That's the focus of Step One.

When You Carry
the Weight of the World

If this were any other weight-loss book, you would not expect Chapter 2 to be about shared energy fields and our interactions with our bodies, emotions, and thoughts. Why am I sending you down a quantum rabbit hole after chocolate-covered carrots? Because this is not a typical weight-loss book. We're going beyond mechanics and into quantum mechanics, into exploring the energy of thoughts and feelings and interactions. It's not just the food that goes in your mouth that makes you fat, or the physical energy you expend that makes you thin. What you take in from the field of energy around you filled with information whizzing around like radio waves affects your weight, too—and this is the thread we've got to look at if you are going to get to the bottom of why you're not losing the weight.

Researchers are still learning about the mind/body/spirit connections, so I can't tell you *exactly* how your weight fluctuations and your mental state are related, but I can suggest some connections. There have been many intriguing scientific discoveries lately that will make the wheels in your mind start turning and will validate what your intuition has already told you: that this weight-loss stuff is more complex than you've been told, and that emotional and mental stress *can* make you gain and retain weight. For instance, did you know that your thoughts and emotions affect you at a *cellular* level?

These complex ideas, which are so different from what most of us have been exposed to in school or in the media, certainly make my head spin, so I'm going to simplify them a bit. I'll start by explaining the nature of the energy field that both surrounds us and includes us (we're each a part of this "fabric" of reality), and how we communicate in ways we can't see, sending information back and forth through the energy field. Then I'll touch on why our thoughts and feelings have energy, and how metabolism works, and then I'll go into why you may never have heard these ideas before. The more you understand the science behind the mind-body connection, the more you'll realize how important it is to do the exercises in this program and why they'll help you stop carrying the "weight of the world."

THE FIELD AND YOU

Just as there is a fabric of your life, there is a fabric of reality that all of us are part of. We all can sense this fabric, or field of energy, although some of us are more aware of it than others. The energy field comprises many types of energy, which is coming from people, animals, plants, the earth, the sun, the planets, and so on; but for simplicity's sake, let's just call it the *electromagnetic field* that we all share.

Even people who don't think of themselves as sensitive can pick up on extremely subtle changes in this energy field. Studies by the Heart-Math Institute, which conducts research and educates people about stress, energy, and the heart, show that our brain waves respond to electromagnetic signals from the heart of a person in the same room with us. If someone is staring at us, we'll almost certainly look up because we sense that person's energy. *Haven't we all had that experience?* Our senses regularly pick up stimuli that can be observed and measured by scientists, but clearly we're also able to pick up the presence of another person, even when we can't see, hear, smell, or touch that person.

Something very subtle is going on. We know we have sensory receptors: the receptors in the inner ear, for example, pick up sound waves and send the information to the brain; the receptors in the skin tell the brain that something's happening—a change in temperature or touch, for instance. Maybe somewhere on our bodies there are sensory receptors we don't know even about. Maybe our sensory receptors are receiving subtle signals that a scientist's instruments can't detect but that our brains notice and register.

Some people insist that they can smell snow, perceive the flicker and sound of fluorescent lights, and even, in cases of a rare condition called *synesthesia*, perceive that sounds have certain colors and shapes. It seems their brains take in and process sensory information differently from the rest of us; they are more sensitive. Remember: dogs have a fantastic, heightened sense of smell, and bats and dolphins have sonar and can perceive solid objects they can't see. It's possible that, early on, humans used to have more acute senses, too, and perhaps some of us have retained that ability, for whatever reason. We just don't have the measurement tools to prove that the person who smells snow isn't making it up.

What if you can pick up on the tension or anger lingering in an empty room after two people have argued in that space? Could the changes in the room's energy field, which a highly intuitive person might pick up on, be perceived and even measured by scientists someday in the future? It wouldn't be the first time people thought "nothing's there" when it actually was. Years ago, surgeons scoffed at the "preposterous notion" that there were tiny little creatures called bacteria that could get into a patient's bloodstream and make him sick if the doctor didn't wash his hands before operating. Thank goodness we figured that one out.

And maybe we simply have areas in our energy field that are open to receive whatever signals come from outside of us—say, we're like radios with our personal energy fields serving as one big antenna. Whatever the nature of our porous boundaries, we pick up signals much like a radio picks up radio waves that convey information and music being broadcast. None of us is immune to changes in the energy field that occur all around us.

FROM ENERGY TO PHYSICAL REALITY:
THE NATURE OF THE "BOND"

When our personal energy field changes, our body responds. Neuro-scientist Candace Pert's pioneering research has shown that whenever we feel an emotion, we also experience an instant physical response: our bodies create molecules called *neuropeptides* that travel through our bloodstream and hook up with receptor cells in the brain, the skin, the stomach, and so on, and they let those cells know what we're feeling. Two of the more well-known peptides are serotonin and endorphins, which, when they meet up with receptor sites, change our mood for the better. There are also peptides that let our cells know we're angry, resentful, or fearful. When the cells in the digestive system receive these peptides, we say, "I feel in my gut that something's wrong"—which is literally true.

The body also responds to thoughts and emotions by releasing hor-mones into the bloodstream. For example, when we're scared or under emotional stress, upset or angry, our adrenal glands release *cortisol*. That's why when someone says something upsetting, we can feel ourselves shak-ing: the body has instantly created the "juice" needed for us to put up a fight or to run away. In fact, our emotional and physical responses hap-pen so quickly that our logical brains may take a few seconds to catch up. (*Wait, what did he just say to me?*) Then, if we start thinking about just how angry or scared we are, the anger is intensified. (*I can't believe he said that! He's a jerk! Who does he think he is? He's always doing this to me.*) We talk ourselves into freaking out and the adrenals pump out more cortisol.

Why do thoughts and emotions, which seem like incredibly subtle energies, have such powerful effects on our bodies? Because physical ob-jects are collections of energy that interact with each other.

At the smallest level of physical reality—the subatomic level—our bodies are not solid, unless we choose to see them that way. If we had far better eyesight, we could see what the most powerful microscopes can: that any solid object, including a human body, is made up of *photons*, or waves of light. These are only shaped into matter, or particles, when they're observed or perceived. If you expect to see a photon, it's a photon.

If you expect to see a particle, well, that smallest unit of reality will oblige and appear as a piece of matter. In other words, *our consciousness—our thoughts and intentions—determine the nature of reality itself.*

These photons, or particles, are constantly vibrating through empty space, so your body is actually made up of quite a lot of air—although it doesn't feel that way when you step on a scale! Now, if you think about anything else that vibrates, like a guitar string, you know that it's easily affected by a vibration outside of it. Play an A string on a guitar, and the A string on a guitar across the room will vibrate in sympathy. Your body works this way, too: you can actually get your heart to entrain to the rhythm of music just by listening to it. Your energy field is not sealed off with solid boundaries; it will always interact with the energy fields around you.

THE MYSTERY OF THE BOND BETWEEN US— AND BETWEEN OUR CELLS

Lynne McTaggart, a science writer and author of *The Intention Experiment* and *The Bond*, points out that we're constantly communicating with the field outside of us and experiencing what she calls "the bond." As she writes:

> Between the smallest particles of our being, between our body and our environment, between ourselves and all of the people with whom we are in contact, between every member of every societal cluster, there is as Bond, a connection so integral and profound that there is no longer a clear demarcation between the end of one thing and the start of another. The world essentially operates, not through the activity of individual things, but in the connection between them—in a sense, in the space between things [*The Bond*].

What else is in this space between things? What's in the dark matter that we find among the stars, planets, and comets? What information is exchanged between me and you, between one starling and another as they fly in unison? What information is exchanged between our cells? Cellular biologist Bruce Lipton upended the world of biology when he discovered that the brain of the cell—the seat of its intelligence—is not in its nucleus, safely ensconced deep inside that cell, but in its membrane, the part of the cell that interacts with everything outside of it. Is it communicating with "the bond," the space between it and the next cell? Is there a vast network of messages being communicated between cells, just as invisible as radio waves when you look into the sky and see nothing moving from transmitter to receiver?

What happens in the space between you and me when one of us creates loving, supportive thoughts and imagines sending them to the other? Researchers at the Institute of Noetic Sciences, in Petaluma, California, conducted an experiment in which they had one member of a couple send loving, healing thoughts to the other, who was in another room, with instruments measuring the response. The recipient experienced changes in heart waves, brain waves, breathing, and blood flow. What's more, another experiment showed that when two people were in separate rooms with their eyes closed, and one was exposed to a flashing light, the other person's brain responded as if it had seen the light, too.

Is this what happens when birds, flocking together, suddenly shift direction simultaneously, then shift back, and back again, in perfect synchronization? The scientists may have theories, but they really don't understand how the birds are communicating with one another instantly, as if they're of one mind. Maybe we are *all* of one mind and just don't realize it! If this is true, then our bodies are responding to a lot more than just our own, personal anger or sadness.

As we're talking about the body's response to emotions, we should also consider the role of thoughts and beliefs. Clearly, thoughts and beliefs can exacerbate emotions, but do they *create* emotions? Or, do we have the emotions and then make sense of them by creating thoughts and beliefs? Or, perhaps there is no real line separating the two. (*I'm furious. Well, no wonder. He just insulted me.*) For people who feel too much, emotions and thoughts are always intertwined.

Obviously, our beliefs can affect our emotions as well. (*He thinks she's better than I am! Boy, that burns me up!*) Our emotions and others' emotions affect our bodies, and so do our personal beliefs—and the beliefs of those around us that we've come to internalize. It seems we *feel* long before we understand what's going on. Our limbic brains experience fear before our prefrontal cortexes can make sense of it all, using words (*Oh, I get what's happening. Hey, I'm not actually being insulted here, so there's no need to feel anger. I'm just misinterpreting his anger as being directed at me.*) That is *not* our instant reaction.

We don't just affect other people with our feelings, thoughts, and beliefs; we also affect physical objects that don't have feelings or emotions (at least, as far as we can tell, they don't). In *The Intention Experiment*, Arizona University professor Dr. Gary Schwartz and Lynne McTaggart describe an interesting experiment they conducted. People in a controlled laboratory setting in London, England, were asked to focus their thoughts on a particular leaf sitting in a lab, thousands of miles away, in Arizona. The subjects had to imagine the leaf glowing. Shortly, the leaf began to emit biophotons that were picked up by a very sensitive camera, while another leaf lying next to it, which was not the object of the subjects' thoughts, remained the same. Similar experiments involving beans and water showed similar results.

So, if thoughts and feelings have such a powerful effect on a leaf, or on water, how much do you suppose your beliefs and emotions, or the thoughts and beliefs you take in from others, affect your cells and organs? For instance, what happens when you think, *I'm fat?* How does your body respond to the belief, *To be a good person, I have to take care of others, no matter how hard the burden is?* Does that get your cortisol running? What if you feel the disapproval of others, believe others think you're fat, or pick up on their beliefs that you're not good enough?

While we're at it, what emotions and thoughts do you hold on to when you hear bad news, like the precariousness of the global financial markets or the 7 billion people on the planet competing for limited resources? How do those emotions and thoughts affect your body?

It's hard to feel confident and to believe you, personally, will be okay when everyone else is telling you that the economy is going to collapse, that you'd better have a basement full of supplies to survive the disaster that's looming. When you're constantly exposed to fearful beliefs—"The whole world is going to pot and we'll be fighting each other over clean drinking water!"—is it possible that your body is responding by storing calories as fat, "just in case"?

Of course, we have some control over our beliefs and, consequently, over our emotions. Let's say we become aware of our fears, and our fear-driven beliefs, and we *consciously* release them (which you'll learn how to do using techniques in this book). When we change our emotions, we change our field of energy and then others who come in contact with that energy entrain themselves to our higher vibration. Have you ever been in a group and felt the fear and contraction other people were experiencing, or, conversely, felt a collective sense of hope and joy? When that happens, you're tuning in to the vibrations of people around you and you are changing your energy field in response to theirs (which is easier than affecting theirs, as you're outnumbered and collective vibration is very strong).

MIRROR NEURONS: I SEE MYSELF IN YOU

About twenty years ago, neuroscientists made a discovery that helped us understand why we experience empathy—why we're able to actually experience someone else's emotions. For example, if I got stung by a bee and yell, "Ouch!" you cringe and actually have a fear reaction—a raising of your own cortisol levels. If you smile, I smile back without even realizing it, and that creates endorphins in my body in response to suddenly feeling your joy as my own. This happens because our brains have something called *mirror neurons* that allow us to imagine ourselves in someone else's shoes.

If I don't have enough mirror neurons, I'll see you smiling but I may not smile in return, unless I stop and think, "Oh, he's smiling. I should probably smile back so he thinks I'm a nice person." I wouldn't actually *experience* your happiness. And when I got stung by that bee, you would know to be polite and express sympathy, but you wouldn't tense up as if you'd been stung yourself. Mirror neurons are believed to be associated not just with empathy but also with our ability to pick up on others' intentions, our sense of self, and our ability to learn language. They probably played an important role in our development of social groups, too. If we didn't feel each other's pain and joy, we might not have become so committed to helping each other, even at risk to ourselves—something necessary for humans to survive in difficult times.

What if those of us who feel too much have more mirror neurons than most people or if our mirror neurons are somehow more sensitive? Maybe people who feel too much have brains that are better able to experience what others are experiencing emotionally. If so, we are taking in more, processing more, and being more sensitive to subtle changes in people's energy fields that are intertwined with ours.

METABOLISM: BEYOND THE SIMPLE EQUATION

Aside from being influenced by what's going on in "the bond," our cells, and our brains, we also experience the effects of something called our *metabolism*, which is our body's process of using the calories we take in. Metabolism is a fairly simple concept: our body burns calories, or units of energy, at a particular rate. We burn more calories when we're engaged in activity; and when we have good muscle tone, we're getting enough quality sleep, and we're managing emotional stress well. That's when our metabolism is fairly high. When we're not doing all those things, our metabolism slows down and our body uses fewer calories to do the same activities it always has, from thinking to moving to digesting. The extra calories are stored as fat, so as we use fewer units of energy, we get fatter.

All of us have a predetermined set point for metabolism, meaning that there are limits to just how much we can speed up our rate of burning calories. For that matter, we also are programmed to have a particular body shape. If we come from ancestors who are short and stocky, there's little we can do to change that basic body shape. Additionally, we're programmed to have our metabolism slow down as we age. It's harder to lose weight as we get older.

However, let's look again at the list of things we can do to affect our metabolism for the better. Two of them are moving more and getting more sleep, which I do want you to do as you move through this program and you've begun to work on managing your empathy. The third is to reduce stress. Is taking on the weight of the world just a teeny bit stressful? And does stress make it hard to get a good night's sleep? Are you seeing some of the threads in the tapestry? By not taking control of your porous boundaries, you're actually lowering your metabolism and using fewer calories. That's going to change as a result of this program.

SO WHY DOESN'T MY DOCTOR KNOW THAT MY FEAR AND FRUSTRATION ARE MAKING ME FAT?

Physicians and scientists all acknowledge a mind-body connection, that our thoughts and feelings affect our immune systems, our hormones, our digestive systems, and so on. Every day, there are new discoveries about the relationships between thoughts, feelings, and physical reality. Even so, many people underestimate just how much thoughts and feelings affect their bodies; they might get to this point in the book and say, "What a bunch of woo-woo nonsense." I get it. But let me explain why the medical community, the media, and most people are just a bit behind on all the evidence for this connection—and why I'm not crazy!

Science has its own rules, and I respect them. We've all benefited greatly from scientific discoveries that came about by following those rules. However, science is a tool for understanding that's also influenced by human weaknesses, like greed, fear, and discomfort with anything that's new and unfamiliar. One of the rules of science is, "Extraordinary claims require extraordinary evidence." That is, what you and I know through experience isn't enough to satisfy a researcher. It takes many research studies, all showing the same results, for scientists to agree that the findings are reliable.

Some of you are old enough to remember how, years ago, many male gynecologists told their female patients, "There's no such thing as PMS. It's all in your head." That was easy for them to say—they hadn't experienced it themselves. And why pay attention to a bunch of women's complaints? Yes, sexism was quite a big factor in preventing research into women's health. Female patients managed not to leap out of their chairs and throttle their doctors for being so obtuse; and eventually, enough people figured out there might be something to this PMS stuff, that it might make sense to research it. Surprise, surprise—women weren't nuts after all, and there *were* physiological reasons for brain fog, mood swings, and cramps. Lesson learned: *just because YOU haven't experienced something doesn't mean it doesn't exist.*

So, if you were to say to a doctor, "Boy, your last patient was really upset before leaving this exam room; I can feel it," your physician might look at you funny, but if enough people made these kinds of observations, scientists might decide that sensing the emotional energy that remains in a room after a person has gone is worth studying. But then scientists would have to find someone willing to invest money in research that would provide the evidence that we're not crazy when we say that emotional energy remains in a physical space after someone has become angry or scared, and that energy can be sensed by highly empathetic people. Why invest money in this research? What's the payoff? Where's the potential for a profitable pharmaceutical drug or procedure that would come out of it? Much of our scientific research is driven by the need for a financial payoff down the road, so there's a lot we don't study simply because there's no money to be made from the potential findings.

These days, when research uncovers new discoveries, it may make the news or be posted on social media and websites, and it may get around much more quickly than years ago. Even so, it takes, on average, *seventeen years* for research to make its way into mainstream clinical practice. If your doctor tells you today about some health treatment that has lots of scientific evidence to back it up, chances are that the treatment was discovered back when DVDs were the latest thing.

So, while you may not have heard about neuropeptides, or the findings of the Intention Experiment, or Dr. Bruce Lipton's groundbreaking work on cell function, these will be common knowledge to the next generation. Meanwhile, it's nice to know that there's some scientific evidence that our experiences as people who feel too much are real!

Knowing that we actually are taking in more energy than others helps us to recognize why we feel overwhelmed so often. The trick is to learn how to have control over our porous boundaries so that we can benefit from them without feeling that we need to curl up in a ball in a dark room with a nice box of chocolates. The Weight Loss for People Who Feel Too Much program has the tools you need to address your empathy overload, so let's get started!

PART TWO

Ready to Go

The Weight Loss for People Who Feel Too Much Program ("Now, That's a Simple Plan I Can Follow!")

You've probably heard of the KISS rule: Keep It Simple, Stupid. I have my own KISS rule for the program—four simple ideas that make up a simple plan for managing your porous boundaries:

- **Kindness.** Be kind to yourself and practice self-compassion.
- **IN-Vizion® Exercises.** Use these special exercises for helping you to manage your difficult emotions.
- **Salt.** Incorporate the healing power of Himalayan salt into your daily life.
- **Simplicity.** Engage in simple eating and simple movement, and maintain a simple energy field (which includes reducing stimulation from the media and from communications technology).

Why is simplicity important? As people who feel too much, we often overcomplicate matters. It's difficult for us to experience emotions without drama, embellishment, agitation, and a sense that we no longer know where we end and others begin. Whenever a strong, upsetting emotion arises, we tend to begin an internal dialogue that keeps that feeling alive: *Of course, I'm angry. I have a right to be! I'm always getting mixed up with people who disrespect me, and this one—well, it's my fault, I should have known better. What was she thinking when she did that? Well, I'll bet I know. I'll bet she was feeling. . . .* Building up the fire of anxiety or anger by throwing gasoline on it is such an ingrained habit that we vacillate between histrionics and withdrawal. We're either in a maelstrom of emotions or we avoid "going there" and looking at our emotions unless we absolutely have to.

And we're not just dealing with our own emotions and inadvertently turning them into wildfires. We're taking on the emotions of everyone else, from the people in line at the bank, to our aunt's stepdaughter who just put an upsetting post on the social media, to our dog who is moping about ever since that encounter with a skunk the day before. We're like a big old sponge that needs wringing out. Rather than confront all that powerful emotion, we take the nearest exit around the scene of our agitation. I'll go into some of our common detours in the last part of this book, but for now, the main one to be aware of is *free eating*.

For people who feel too much, eating should always be contained. It needs to have a beginning, middle, and end. Otherwise, we graze to ground ourselves and eat more than we need to—and most of those extra calories come from foods we should be limiting in the first place. We like to make sure we've got stashes of food so that wherever we are, we can instantly satisfy our need *to feel present in our bodies.*

Maybe you nibble on this and that to keep your mood stable throughout the morning, then when lunchtime comes around, you're not really hungry so you skip the meal and feel proud of your willpower until about 4:00, when that craving for sweets, fats, salts, and processed carbohydrates hits hard. Then you end up plowing through four servings of the nearest packaged treat. Instead of using food for nourishment, and meals as a time to focus on your body's needs, *you're using food for mood management.*

Another common detour for people who feel too much is overcomplicating our eating habits and goals. Because our emotions are swirling about like the objects outside of Dorothy Gale's window in *The Wizard of Oz*, we try to take control of everyone and everything, especially our eating and our weight. We get enslaved by calorie counts and scales, or we try to justify overeating by gorging on "healthy" cookies and chips and fool ourselves into thinking that if we obsess over what we consume, we'll be just fine. We use dieting itself as a detour, we don't manage our emotions, we binge out of a feeling of desperation, then we beat ourselves up. The mad back-and-forth between free eating and obsession over eating has to stop, and this program will show you how.

KINDNESS

Remember earlier when I was talking about how I am not a drill sergeant, and I don't want you to "battle" your weight? Many people who feel too much were taught from earliest childhood that if they want to get something done, they have to be tough, and even brutal, as they push forward. As it turns out, research shows that this is *not* the best way to approach weight loss. Showing kindness toward yourself, having self-compassion, is more effective than willpower when it comes to sticking to your eating goals. In fact, willpower can be depleted quickly; exercising willpower uses glucose (sugar), which might explain why, when you're feeling stressed by dieting, you start to crave sugar. And I'm sure you won't be surprised to hear that social stress makes it harder to exercise willpower. However, getting enough quality sleep and being in a good mood boost willpower, as do eating well and getting movement. In short, research shows that well-being makes it easier to resist temptation.

So, no more battling, no more self-loathing, no more beating yourself up over what you ate: all of that is standing in the way of your getting to the root of your weight problem and your disordered eating.

One of the key ways to be kind to yourself is by affirming your worth and your love for yourself. A fantastic means of doing this is through the Emotional Freedom Technique, or EFT, which you will be doing daily throughout the program. I discovered this technique many years ago, when I saw a friend of mine tapping on the side of her hand and her collarbone. She was doing this while quietly saying an affirmation, and I asked her, What are you doing? She told me she was doing a technique she learned that was a form of "emotional acupuncture"—a tapping exercise accompanied by specific verbal affirmations. I was interested, so I asked her to show me. (I had had a particularly difficult day and had argued with a family member, and was feeling overwhelmed.) I did what she told me, and within minutes I began to feel an obvious relief!

Yet, like many of the techniques I explored that were practiced by the alternative healing arts community, I was more of a tourist in some exotic foreign land; I didn't stick around long enough to really learn the lay of the land. I was curious, and I continued to do the EFT, but I didn't put the puzzle pieces together. I hadn't realized how EFT could help with weight release until I discovered a book called *EFT for Weight Loss*, written by one of the pioneers of EFT, Gary Craig. So, I decided to see if it would work for me. When I added EFT to my repertoire of weight-loss techniques, I was amazed how my craving for sugar just went bye-bye after a month of using EFT. Then I decided to add a version of EFT to my classes for the Weight Loss for People Who Feel Too Much program, and some of the participants said the technique helped calm their anxiety.

Although still considered in its experimental phase, Emotional Freedom Technique is being practiced by personal-development coaches and energy-medicine specialists worldwide. The documentary film on EFT, *The Tapping Solution*, features endorsements by many reputable experts in the medical community, from psychologists and biologists to neurologists, as well as leading authors in the personal-development field, such as Jack Canfield and Cheryl Richardson. If you experiment with EFT yourself, you may very well find it a fun and easy way to calm down the emotional overwhelm that plagues people who feel too much.

In doing EFT, you work with acupuncture meridians, stimulating them in order to loosen any blocks in the flow of vital energy (also known as *chi*). Blocks in the flow of energy can cause emotional symptoms, such as feeling ashamed, unmotivated, or resentful, or physical symptoms, such as a disturbance in your blood circulation, a tightness in your muscles, or a hormone imbalance. When your energy is running freely and smoothly, as it's meant to do, your emotions and your physical systems respond by running freely and smoothly as well.

Simply put, for EFT, use your index and middle finger to tap lightly on particular spots on your body as you speak affirmations, such as "No matter that I've chosen to eat foods that are not the best for me, I deeply love and respect myself," and "No matter that I'm imperfect and I devoured two cupcakes, I deeply and completely love and respect myself." The tapping slows the heart rate by increasing your body's production of the calming biochemicals GABA (an amino acid), serotonin (a neurotransmitter), and opioids, and awakens your body's ability to both calm the area of the brain that experiences anxiety and help you to reabsorb cortisol, the stress hormone. It may even alter gene expression and boost immunity.

The affirmation works similarly to cognitive behavioral therapy techniques, in that you're both acknowledging your problem and putting it into perspective. In the first half of the affirmation, you admit to the behavior, thought, or quality that you'd prefer not to think about. This draws your attention to the problem and the block you want to dissolve. In the second half of the affirmation, you acknowledge your deep, unconditional love and respect for yourself.

For the EFT tapping, use your index and middle finger to tap gently on your body at these acupuncture points:

- the middle of your forehead
- the spot on your brow ridge just above your nose and slightly to the right
- the spot on your brow ridge just above your nose and slightly to the left
- your right cheekbone
- your left cheekbone
- the space between your nose and your upper lip
- the middle of your chin
- your heart
- your collarbone, a few inches to the right of your heart
- your collarbone, a few inches to the left of your heart
- under your right arm, halfway down your rib cage

- under your left arm, halfway down your rib cage
- on the fleshy part of your right hand's outer ridge (the Karate Chop Point [KC] where you would do a karate chop)
- on the fleshy part of your left hand's outer ridge

Say your affirmations while you do the entire tapping sequence. Each time you recite the affirmation, tap repeatedly on the acupuncture point. Work through all the EFT points, using the same affirmation or several different affirmations. All your affirmations should follow the format I described earlier: acknowledge the problem and affirm your deep love and respect for yourself.

Pay attention to how you feel when you're tapping. Do any emotions arise? You can do a tapping sequence to acknowledge that feeling. And you may find other layers beneath the ones you begin with. After you've finished tapping, you will probably feel calmer, and you'll sense that you've released some emotions. At first, you may need to do two or three rounds of tapping on the same topic to feel a difference, but as you tap more, you will loosen your emotions more quickly.

With some practice, EFT can take only a minute or two. Instead of checking your social media, go into a bathroom stall or off to an empty room and do your EFT. I do mine at my desk if or when something triggers me. Granted, it does look a little weird in public; but if I need to do a tapping round when I'm out, I only use the KC point on the side of my left hand. Tap-tap-tap becomes second nature to you as you shift your mood and stay in the moment.

Doing EFT is one way of many introduced in this program to be kind to yourself and to commit to a new way of managing your emotional energy. Another, most important way is to speak your truth, which is the focus of Step One, discussed in Chapter 4. The safest place to speak your truth is in a journal, so many journaling exercises have been included in the program. Most important, as you will learn later, you should have not one, but two journals. One is for what I refer to as the "Dumping Grounds"; the other is for "Solutions and Insights." Starting with Step

Two, discussed in Chapter 5, these journals will be used to reinforce your positive feelings and thoughts about yourself, and to help you separate out the passages that are laden with painful feelings you want to release. Later on in the program, you'll learn about venting to your journal and then performing a ritual I call "sorting through and dumping the garbage." When you do this, you'll free yourself of the weight imposed by those strong emotions connected to your "garbage."

Every day of the program, you'll do a little bit of journal writing in the morning and evening, answering just a few questions. During the active weeks, you'll be answering two to three other questions as part of the "daily journal writing" exercise. In addition, you'll journal about your responses to the exercises you do—and any time you feel you need to speak your truth.

Throughout the program, every morning, you'll write down your answers to these questions:

What is my intention?
What do I want to experience today?

Every night just before bed, you'll journal your answer to these questions:

How did I do? (Did you have an off-day and if so, why? What happened?)
What is one thing I did that I can be happy about and proud of?
What is one thing I'm grateful for?

Even on your worst days, you will find something you did right, even if it was to follow through on your commitment to write in your journal. As for naming one thing you're grateful for, I'm not making an idle request. According to research by Robert A. Emmons, of the University of California at Davis, and Michael E. McCullough, of the University of Miami, regularly acknowledging what you're grateful for will make you happier, healthier, and more optimistic.

In addition to your morning and evening journaling, you'll have daily journal questions to answer during each active week of the program.

The daily questions and many of the exercises in this program will stir up emotions, so be sure to set aside a time when you'll feel comfortable accessing those feelings. Devote at least 20 minutes a day to your journal writing, and be sure not to skip the morning and bedtime daily writing, either. It's really important to set your intention for each day, and to end the day by affirming something positive you've accomplished.

THE IN-VIZION PROCESS

Inspired by Swiss psychologist Carl Jung's active imagination method of accessing the wisdom of the unconscious, I created the IN-Vizion Process, now the signature process I teach to Weight Release Energetix® coaches who work with clients in need of personal coaching while they follow the weight-loss program described in this book. While working with a coach is helpful, you can—and are meant to—do this daily and as often as you need to on your own. The versions of it I have included here are an integral part of the weight-loss program and essential for your success.

Even more important to this program than my suggestion about using EFT, the IN-Vizion Process is designed specifically to give you quick relief from empathy overload and enable a state of mind called *neutral observation*. The process bypasses analytical logic and reason, to move you rapidly out of personalized, highly charged emotional states and into the domain of the creative right brain, imagination, and intuition. IN-Vizion works by incorporating intention, guided visualization, and active imagination to help you tap into, dialogue with, and interact with your unconscious dreaming mind in order to reprogram your subconscious emotionally patterned mind.

Although the actual model of the mind is much more complex, think of the levels of consciousness as threefold. The "thinking mind" is where you actively think thoughts that come with actions like reading and comprehending this book. That's your *conscious mind*. Then, there's the level of the mind that is programmed to make your heart beat, and where everything you learn about the world is recorded, especially repetitive reinforced experiences, so that you react to stimuli automatically. That's your *subconscious mind*. And then there's the vast reservoir of the mind that contains the memory of everything you have ever experienced. This is the *unconscious*—the dreaming mind. It also taps into a fourth *collective unconscious*, where all the experiences ever had by all of humanity are purported to exist.

The unconscious is the reservoir of imagination that first becomes activated by the IN-Vizion Process. It's almost a little like dreaming while you're awake! Ever heard the saying "A picture speaks a thousand words"? The unconscious and the subconscious communicate in pictures and images, not in words. And it is the ability to imagine in images that allows you to access information you can't get at by thinking in words. Most of what you need to know is hidden deep inside you, just like buried treasure. The IN-Vizion Process helps you find the gold!

When you use the IN-Vizion Process, you start with the intention of discovering a landscape that represents the content hidden in your sub-conscious mind, below your active thinking mind. These pictures and images are delivered to you by the unconscious—the dreaming—mind. Deep down, if you are asked to describe the environment of your state of mind by using metaphors of the natural world, you will know whether your emotions are an arid, lonely desert or a cluttered attic. You may not be able to articulate that feeling, but your subconscious mind will express it in the form of an image if you ask it to. Remember, the deeper layers of the mind speak in pictures, not words!

Then, when you have the image of the landscape, and you connect to the act of "seeing it" as outside of you, you can begin to meditate by clearing your mind of thoughts and focusing only on your breathing. Once you are aware of the landscape, you can experience your emotions as an objective observer might, instead of feeling that you are lost in an emotional experience that's beyond your control. After all, you can always depart from a landscape.

When you do the IN-Vizion Process exercises, the emotions you feel may be strong, but you'll be able to handle them and learn from your experience of them. You'll find that, over time, you don't keep ending up in the same distressing landscape—or when you do, you don't stay long because you easily walk out of it.

Throughout the weight-loss program, I provide you with several IN-Vizion Process exercises you can use at any time to gain insights about yourself. You can also download many recorded versions of the IN-Vizion Process, accompanied with original music some of which has binaural beats brain-wave technology imbedded; visit my website www.colette baronreid.com/weightloss.

You can also find a Weight Release Energetix certified coach listed on my website, should you want help with this program. I introduced this IN-Vizion Process in my book *The Map: Finding the Magic and Meaning in the Story of Your Life*. As a highly effective technique, it can be applied to any situation where you require a perceptual shift in order to gain clarity and objectivity when faced with a highly charged reactive emotional state of mind. The process is the foundation for all the vigorous certification training I have developed for my coaching institute, The Master Intuitive Coach Institute; to learn more, go to www.micicoach.com.

There are many exercises in the IN-Vizion Process that can help a person who feels too much, especially around issues with food. The Landscape of Your Hunger exercise (see below) is one of my favorites, and one that will help you connect to your inner wisdom about food and your body.

THE LANDSCAPE OF YOUR HUNGER

Before starting to eat a meal or snack, pay attention to your hunger. Close your eyes and take several slow, deep breaths to quiet your mind. Don't try to analyze what you're experiencing. Simply allow your subconscious mind to show you images that will help you process your emotions, as directed. Your imagination is an active part of your consciousness, and when asked for a representation of your state of mind, it's just dying to talk to you—not in words, but in pictures. The deeper mind speaks in imagery and metaphor.

Continue breathing slowly and feeling your hunger. Let your subconscious mind show you a landscape that represents your hunger. Ask yourself:

What is this landscape?

What are its features?

Sense whether the food you're about to eat enhances or detracts from this landscape. For instance, does this food intensify the weather conditions? Do the storms rage harder? Does the rain fall in sheets? Does the desert sun become stronger and hotter?

If you eat this food, how will the landscape change? Will eating this food bring into your vision another landscape nearby that you can travel to? What is that landscape? Do you wish to go there?

Will eating this food take you from this landscape to that one?

Now imagine there is a place where you can plant this food as if it were a seed that will sprout and grow. If you plant this food, what will grow from the seed? Is it something you want to grow?

Now ask yourself:

Do I want to eat this food right now?

What do I hunger for at this moment?

Listen for the answer.

Journal about this experience and the insights you gained.

~~~~~~

Keep in mind that whatever you experience in these places in your mind, you're always in charge. No matter how emotionally painful the truth is that they reveal, you are safe. In fact, a great way to create that sense of safety is to use the IN-Vizion Process to let your subconscious mind suggest a landscape that will serve as your sanctuary. This sanctuary is one you can consciously escape to through a visualization process or by using the IN-Vizion Process.

What might you find in that safe haven that could help you feel at peace? The following exercise will help you discover an inner landscape that is a quiet resting place, one that will show itself again whenever you wish to go to this imaginary place.

DISCOVER YOUR INNER SANCTUARY

Take a few deep, long, slow breaths and focus on your inhalation and exhalation. Let your mind and body relax. Ask yourself,

Where am I?

Wait for your mind to show you a landscape. Notice the features of the land and your relationship to it. Ask yourself,

Who is looking at this landscape?

Who is observing it?

Pay particular attention to how you are experiencing the observer role.

What does it feel like to look, to observe, to be the one looking?

Notice what your relationship to this landscape is now. Are you in a safe spot on that landscape, observing what's going on?

Feel your power to move out of this landscape. You are in charge. Survey the landscape for a means to escape. What do you see? Ask yourself,

Where would I like to go next?

Allow a new landscape to reveal itself. Observe how your means to escape can take you there. Do you see a bridge? A bird that can carry you?

Use your power to escape to your sanctuary.

Notice what you feel, what you see, what you hear. What

textures are you experiencing? What do you feel beneath your feet? Let all the sensory details of your sanctuary come into your awareness, making you feel calm, rejuvenated, and peaceful. Be in harmony with this landscape.

Once you enter your sanctuary, allow your imagination to show yourself as a 4-year-old. Smile, and imagine your heart opening wide with love and acceptance to this innocent little child, and say whatever you need to help her or him feel safe, then hug and breathe deeply, connecting to the power of committing to loving and protecting. This can be a powerful way of healing childhood hurts without analyzing any of the details.

When you are ready, open your eyes and return slowly to ordinary consciousness.

~~~~~~

Whenever you do an IN-Vizion exercise, you'll find it can be really helpful to write about the experience in your journal. For one thing, you can see how your inner landscapes evolve over time, in detail and impact. Your subconscious mind will respond beautifully as your unconscious, or dreaming mind, activates its symbolic language to speak to you about how you're doing and where you're headed. The subconscious is reprogrammed every time you do the same thing, over and over again. Bringing yourself out of the desert and into the sunny and lush garden in your imagination makes it easier to do that in your everyday life.

SALT

Years ago, I noticed that when I lived by the ocean, and swam in it or walked alongside it regularly, it was easier to let go of the emotional weight I was carrying. It was easier to maintain my weight and my equilibrium. It didn't make sense that the ocean was somehow affecting me, but my intuition told me it was. Then I met a classical Feng Shui instructor and Reiki master who kept bowls of salt water in the room she worked in. I asked her what the water was for, and she told me that in traditional Feng Shui, pure salts remove toxins from your energetic environment. *Hmmm, could that be why the ocean had such an effect on me when I lived near it?*

As it turns out, when you heat unprocessed salt like Himalayan salt or put it in water, the molecules that have been held together by electromagnetic energy split apart. The sodium molecules release positive ions, and the chloride crystals release an even larger number of ions—only these are negative. In this case, "negative" is good because negative ions cause more oxygen to flow to our brains, making us more alert. They also remove small particles from the air. These particles can irritate the body when they're inhaled (all that dust that gathers around your electronic equipment is attracted to the positive ions sent out by televisions, computers, and the like). An overabundance of positive ions in the electromagnetic field zaps our energy and makes us feel sluggish or fatigued, or cause headaches. Negative ions are believed to affect serotonin levels in our brains; research suggests that people who have thin boundaries (that's us!) are especially sensitive to changes in the ionization in the environment.

To change the ionization in the electromagnetic field around you, you can use heated Himalayan salt lamps, or place a bowl of highly concentrated rock salt water (half a bowl of salt, just covered barely with water) around you (keep it away from pets, who might lap up the water, and change the water at the end of each day). There are also specially designed heated beds covered in salt that you can lie on, which are available in some spas or for purchase. Make or purchase salt scrubs using Himalayan salts; oils such as almond, jojoba, or grapeseed; and perhaps some essential oils as well, to use on your skin to slough off your day. Of course, if you do live near the ocean, or a natural hot spring that has salt and minerals in it, swim or soak in the water when you can, or at least visit it and breathe in the salty air.

Recipe for Happy Himalayan Salt Scrub

This simple recipe is a wonderful, aromatic scrub that has all the benefits of changing ionization, which helps people who feel too much remain calmer and less stressful. This is a lovely scrub you can use on your hands, feet, and all over your body. And, I feel happy when I use it, so I hope you will, too!

Fill a glass pickling jar two-thirds full with medium-grind Pink Himalayan salt. Then fill one-third of the jar with good-quality Apricot Kernel Oil and Jojoba Oil (see Note).

Add 30 drops of Sweet Orange Pure Aromatherapy Oil.

Add 10 drops of Peppermint Aromatherapy Oil.

Add 10 drops of Lavender Aromatherapy Oil.

Note: It's very easy to find Apricot Kernel Oil and Jojoba Oil at a health food store or a store that sells massage oil. You can use a blend like I do, or choose one or the other. Do not use baby oil or any pre-scented oils.

You can play around with the aromatherapy oils according to your preference.

SALT BATHS

I find the most powerful way to incorporate the health benefits of pure salt into my life is to take a bath with Himalayan salt, along with some essential oils every afternoon at 4:00 P.M., or at some time shortly afterward. Because I work from home as a writer, it's easy for me to do this, especially when I'm under a lot of stress. While I am in the bath, I always use the IN-Vizion Process and sometimes the Emotional Freedom Technique.

This is an enjoyable part of managing my porous boundaries, and I highly recommend that you incorporate it into *your* routine to feel the full benefit of the Weight Loss for People Who Feel Too Much program. Positive changes occur in any energy field when you heat natural salt.

Ritualistic salt baths *will* help you better manage your porous boundaries and avoid becoming overwhelmed emotionally.

A high-quality, natural salt in a hot bath will create plenty of negative ions, as well as contribute to a balanced pH in your body and offer relief of oxidative stress. Pure Himalayan salt also has many minerals that your body needs and will absorb from your bath. This is the salt I recommend, and the only one I use, although any natural unprocessed salt will do the trick. The salt bath can also contain a bit of Epsom salts, or magnesium sulfate, which helps reduce inflammation and relax you. You can find Epsom salts at any drugstore.

I have many favorite aromatherapy blends. Add to the bath the following essential oils for aromatherapy: six drops each of lavender oil (for calming), grapefruit or rosemary oil (for detoxification), and orange oil (a natural analgesic). The bath is an important ritual, so remain in it long enough to feel your energy shift—10 to 20 minutes. Use the Emotional Freedom Technique while saying your affirmations. Afterward, don't let anyone else use the bathwater, which will now contain the energy garbage of your day. You can use it to flush your toilet if you're conserving water. Then, when you get dressed, put on new clothes. Place the old ones, which carry the energy of all the people and places you've interacted with all day, in the hamper.

Why do a bath at 4:00 P.M.? Because about eight to ten hours after waking up, we're most vulnerable to becoming overwhelmed by our empathy and likely to take a detour. It's also when our blood pressure naturally peaks. I know many of you are at work or in school at 4:00 P.M. and won't be able to do the bath until you get home. In that case, use a spritzer of a mild concentration of salt water with the aromatherapy oils to spray yourself and the area immediately around you (do this in the bathroom, not near computers!). Take off one piece of clothing if you can—a sweater, a bracelet, anything that can ritually represent the shedding of your day. Later, when you're at home, you can do the full salt bath ritual.

Many people who feel too much are not used to taking time to nurture themselves. So, you might be feeling some resistance to a daily Himalayan salt bath, even though it will only take you twenty minutes. The people who have done best on this weight-loss program did the baths every day, incorporating EFT into the ritual. So I strongly encourage you to push past that resistance. If you do skip a bath or two, pay attention to how you feel that night, before you go to bed. I think you will see how beneficial the baths are for your ability to manage your porous boundaries. And, it's only for the duration of the program that I suggest that you do the bath regularly. Try committing to a minimum 10 minutes a day for just one week. I know you will see the benefits and will want to keep doing it!

Himalayan Salt Crystals

When you do your salt bath or prepare a salt water spritz, it's important not to use table salt, kosher salt, or other impure processed salts. You should use pure Himalayan salt crystals because this is the purest salt of all. It doesn't contain pollutants as Dead Sea salt or regular salts do (and the latter are highly processed). What's more, it contains many minerals that are naturally present in our body when it's at optimal health. See the Recommended Reading and Resources section of this book for information on where to buy Himalayan salts. Also, I suggest you use Himalayan salts instead of any other salt for sprinkling on food. I present updated information on all of this on my website, www.colettebaronreid.com/weightloss. And, I share everything I find as I discover more amazing things that help people who feel too much release the excess weight they wear, both literally and figuratively!

SIMPLICITY

This program is designed to keep you from detouring into an obsession with food, weight, or exercise and to prevent you from becoming overstimulated, overwhelmed, and stressed out, all of which set you up for disordered eating. The program includes the following dos and don'ts:

- don't weigh yourself
- do move your body every day but don't feel pressured to "exercise"
- do avoid media so you can keep your emotional field uncluttered
- do eat three meals and two snacks a day, avoiding foods that you know trigger disordered eating for you

DON'T WEIGH YOURSELF!

Let's start with your weight. Go ahead and weigh yourself once before starting the program and once at the end. If you feel strongly about wanting to get a sense of where you are halfway through, get weighed at the doctor's office or in front of a kind friend who will write down the number and tell you whether you have lost or maintained your weight. I stand in front of the scale at the doctor's office, facing away from it, and I ask only to be told if I am maintaining a healthy weight or if there is any change from my last visit. I know approximately how much I weigh based on how my clothes fit me. Not everyone is scale-centric, but many of you are. In the past, I would decide whether my entire day was good or a disaster, based on the number on my scale. If that sounds like you, don't reward or torture yourself by getting on it during this program.

So, if you own a scale, hide it in the back of your closet or in the garage. If you start worrying about whether you've lost any weight, stop what you're doing in that moment, close your eyes, and say to yourself, "I love my body. I love you, body! Every inch of you is divine. I accept you and love you just as you are. Thank you for being my protection. You are perfect, and I am safe."

MOVE YOUR BODY EVERY DAY

During the eight weeks of this program, it's important to keep your body moving, but you don't have to commit to a strenuous exercise regime.

In fact, many of you may have a condition called adrenal exhaustion, owing to stress, and if you do too rigorous exercise you'll actually cause more stress to your adrenal glands and wipe yourself out for a day or two with fatigue.

You'll learn more about adrenals and adrenal fatigue later in the book, and be given some more guidance on how to work healthy movement into your life, but for now, just know that you shouldn't feel you absolutely need to start working out like a fiend at the gym. I'm sure you're relieved about that! Having said that, it is contradictory to the program to sit all day long—and it's terrible for your circulation of vital fluids and for your muscles and stamina. You must move to move the energy—you will not experience the relief from empathy overload when you are sedentary.

As you clean up your diet and start untwisting the tangled necklaces in the jewelry box of your emotions, you'll have more energy and you can begin thinking about ways to get more exercise. For the next eight weeks, if possible, get some movement outdoors. Sunshine helps your body make vitamin D and serotonin, the latter which is a feel-good neurotransmitter your body and your mind really needs. Just spending five minutes walking or exercising outdoors can improve your mood.

Movement is especially important when you're feeling angry or anxious. Try just a short, brisk walk, a quick swim, some yoga moves, a few minutes spent dancing vigorously to your favorite songs, or a session on an active video game, such as Wii Fit or X-Box Kinnect games, which require that you get up and move. Strong emotions dissipate more easily when you move your body. Physical exercise is proven to improve the emotional well-being of everyone, as it releases the excess energies accumulated throughout the day.

AVOID MEDIA

As I pointed out earlier, because of technology most of us are *so much more* connected to other people than ever before. It's very hard to get through the day without being exposed to someone's anger, cruelty, or suffering, unless you take a break from television and social media. Your emotional field can get cluttered very quickly with all the negative emotions you're typically exposed to. For the duration of this weight-loss program, avoid as much as possible all television, the news, the Internet, social media, and most magazines (especially gossipy ones). If you play inactive video games or online games of any sort to detour around your own emotions or to stimulate you, stay away from them, too, for the next eight weeks. Dancing, yoga, or exercise video games are okay, but inactive games suck you into acquiring virtual points, livestock, and party invitations and into ignoring the difficult feelings you have to examine.

I know there's a lot going on, and you might feel it's important to stay informed about the news, but if you can't take a total break from the media, then at least avoid visual images, which usually pack a bigger emotional punch than words. And avoid emotionally upsetting stories you don't absolutely have to read, such as the doom-and-gloom pieces on financial blunders and world political situations. Stick with reading good news that will put a smile on your face and make you feel hopeful. When you've completed this program and have established good habits for managing your porous boundaries, then you can start putting media back into your life again. Trust me—you'll be surprised at how little it mattered that you missed eight weeks or so of the media.

EAT THREE MEALS AND TWO SNACKS A DAY

Eat mostly fresh, organic (when you can), plant-based foods that will keep you sated instead of feeling deprived or hungry. At the same time, make sure you quiet the noisy food that stimulates an emotional response. You don't have to measure anything, or worry about what foods you mix at a meal, or avoid certain foods for the first week, or anything like that. That said, I know you want more details, so let me explain a little bit about how to eat simply and healthfully, ignoring the calls of noisy food, eating mindfully, and making detours.

Noisy Food and How to Shut It Up

We all have foods that stimulate a strong emotional response. We tend to crave them physically, but we can crave them emotionally, too, because of their associations. When you're feeling sad or melancholy, as well as physically sluggish, you might crave sugar, but what you really crave is the cookie bars you used to make with your grandmother. Or, you're not satisfied indulging in several pieces of salty pizza when you have a taste for salt; you want to get those slices from the pizzeria where you and your friends used to hang out back when you were in college and were filled with excitement and enthusiasm about what the future would hold. Or, like me, you may have not felt the real connection to your mother when you were younger and food, especially sweets, give you that sense of false nourishment that you connect with the idea of being nurtured emotionally.

Noisy foods call to us when we're not managing our emotions and are deeply seductive when we're in empathy overload and need to feel comforted. They provide a temporary yet powerful sensual escape that we later regret. It's really important that we people who feel too much don't eat for entertainment or emotional sustenance. Enjoy your food, by all means, but don't make it the primary source of your enjoyment. Don't reach for the bag of treats when you really need to reach for your shoes and your phone, and call a friend who will go on a casual walk with you. Sound easy? It's not at first, but with time it gets better and better. Those noisy foods *will* stop yapping at you.

Now, there are also foods that are *literally* noisy. They make your body rumble and grumble with gas, bloating, and indigestion, and make it cry out to you, "Please, I'm so tired! Let me take a nap or zone out on the sofa!" These foods tend to be comfort foods that are too taxing for your system to process, but the pleasure of having them in your mouth distracts you from the discomfort of having them go through your gastro-intestinal system minutes or hours later. Are there any foods you know you'll regret eating but which you indulge in anyway because you can't resist them? As you become more mindful of the foods you're ingesting and how they interact with your body and affect you overall, these foods will be less of a temptation for you.

What is equally important as avoiding these detour foods is the way in which you refer to them. Those foods are not bad or evil. If you label them that way, it makes them even more seductive. All food is just food.

We learn here how to love ourselves to decide which foods will be best for us and which are not the best choices. You can have any food you choose to eat. It's important just to be aware that there are consequences. For example if you know that when you eat cereal you immediately want to overeat it, choosing to eat it may lead to overeating it. I love ice cream. I eat ice cream when I am in a stable mood and once in a while, and always as something I have chosen to eat. Total deprivation isn't the answer, either. If I'm stressed, however, one ice cream cup could easily turn into a large tub before I know it. As for alcohol, I don't touch it—ever. You will find your way with this as you get honest with yourself.

Mindful Eating

Do you eat so much, so quickly, that you're uncomfortably full afterward? Do you eat in a frenzy when you're overcome with a strong emotion, then regret your binge later? Or, are you utterly clueless about how much you eat and how often you're putting food in your mouth?

Mindful eating means being fully present while you're eating instead of having your mind going in seventeen different directions while your food disappears before you. To eat mindfully, you've got to have boundaries to your eating, as I said. Once a meal is over, and the plate or bowl is empty, that's the end. No free eating!

As you begin this program, it's important to pay attention to your eating habits. To do this, you might want to measure how much food fits on one of your plates or in one of your bowls—some bowls actually hold three or four servings of a food, which is great if you fill it with broccoli, not so great if you fill it with pasta. If you're going to eat some chips, take a moment as you stand before them and determine what size portion you want for yourself. Read the label and you might realize you don't want to eat any given how much fat and salt they contain (and beware of labels with misleading serving sizes—please, who eats a half dozen potato chips?).

Once you determine your portion size, place that amount on a plate or napkin, close up the food container, and put it away. You don't actually have to measure food portions (as I said, it's too easy for people who feel too much to start obsessing over these things!). Then again, if you're a person who considers a pound of hamburger or a mega muffin a "just right" portion, it might be a good idea to get some measuring cups to get used to reasonable healthy food portions. In many countries, portion sizes have ballooned over the years. We've become used to bottles of soda pop or servings of salty snacks that are 50 to 60 percent larger than they were thirty years ago. As you get further into building skills to manage your porous boundaries and your emotions, it will become easier to choose, and stick to, smaller portion sizes instead of heading off to the couch with your supersized bag of munchies.

When you eat mindfully, you focus on the food and your body's experience of it. If you tend to eat meals alone, it's understandable that you might want to switch on the TV or watch some online videos to keep yourself entertained while you're eating and keep your mind off your desire for friends or family to sit around a table with you. Did you know that when you eat while watching television, you consume more calories? In fact, women who watch three to four hours of television a day are twice as likely to be obese as women who watch for an hour a day. When you get together with other people to break bread, as they say, you can create a sense of community that would satisfy you much more than watching another reality show or eating a huge plate full of food.

The rule in this weight-loss program is simply to eat when you're hungry, stop when you're full. To do that, you have to be mindful of your hunger signals and stick with a simple plan for eating that prevents dips in blood sugar levels. For the next eight weeks, you will eat three meals and two snacks. Now, there's some flexibility to this rule depending on what your body needs. One of my clients has two light meals for breakfast—some protein and fruit when she gets up and a snack with fiber and whole grains a couple of hours later. Whatever works for you, go for it—but it's very important that you *never* skip a meal. If you do, you're fooling yourself—you're going to eat that meal anyway, just when you're absolutely famished owing to low blood sugar and far more likely to overeat. Then you will probably consume the very foods you're trying to avoid (the noisy ones that scream, "Enough already! You're hungry and you deserve to eat! Take a big handful!"). Be mindful of your body's needs and plan to be around healthful food when you're inevitably going to get hungry. Then have your snack or meal, on a plate. Enjoy it, clean up when you're done, and don't mindlessly scan the refrigerator to see if there's anything else you might want.

On this plan, it's important not to deprive yourself. If you're used to eating a whole chocolate bar every day, don't set a goal of eating no chocolate whatsoever. You'll miss it so much that you'll be tempted to binge. Plan on having perhaps two squares of chocolate a day, or a half a bar twice a week. If you suddenly feel you need to have chocolate you haven't planned for as part of your three meals and two snacks, stop for a moment and ask yourself, *What am I really hungry for? What do I want right now?* You might be surprised to see that when you ask yourself these questions, you will very likely not want that chocolate after all. The real answer will rarely be "a giant chocolate bar."

Everyone is different—our blood types are different, our body shapes are different, our food preferences are different—and you may do better on one food plan than on another. However, what we people who feel too much have in common is that we use food to ground ourselves because *we have too much of our own feelings jumbled up with what we pick up from the environment.* For us, food needs to find its proper place in our lives, and the kind of food we eat matters a great deal.

How to Eat: A Primer

We all know how to eat: it's instinctual, really (well, maybe not eating artichoke leaves—that takes some training). What we don't know is how to eat healthfully. Crazy though it may sound, I'm going to attempt to reteach you how to eat.

Step One. Sit down. We're all busy and on the go much of the time, but you can't eat mindfully if you're walking, standing over a sink, or driving.

Step Two. Make sure your food is contained. As I said, don't worry about portion sizes for now. Just make sure that you're not eating from a big container or an overfilled plate with the intention of eating until you're no longer hungry, or you will eat more than you intend to eat. There was a fascinating study done on unsuspecting subjects who ate from a soup bowl that they didn't realize was being refilled from tubing underneath the bowl and table. Rather than listening to their hunger signals, they let their eyes tell them whether they needed to eat more.

If you were a member of the clean plate club as a child, and felt keenly that it was your personal obligation to make up for all those people starving over in some other country by listening to Mom and eating every morsel on your plate, you will have to let go of that old thinking and start listening to your body's signals about how much food to eat.

Step Three. Turn off the TV and other distractions. Don't eat while talking on the phone, watching TV, or surfing the Internet. It will distract you from how much you are eating and whether what you're eating is what your body needs.

Step Four. Breathe and focus. After serving yourself a snack or meal, take five or six long, deep breaths. Pay attention to how you feel. Are you agitated and responding to noisy food, or are you calm and responding to your body's need for nourishment? You will know beyond a shadow of a doubt if the food is okay for you to eat or not. Listen to your intuition. Taking several slow breaths helps calm your system and any strong emotions, and gets you in touch with your body's divine intelligence, which will tell you what you're truly hungry for. If you're about to eat a food that you realize you don't want, you can mindfully choose not to eat it after all or to exchange it for something your body wants to eat—and you can make this choice without drama.

Step Five. Be grateful. Before you pick up your fork, take a moment to be grateful for the nourishing food in front of you. Imagine where that food came from and how it came to your table. Be grateful for the farmer, the workers who harvested the food, and all those who handled it with integrity before it came to you. Imagine the rich soil, the sunlight, and the rain that gave life to the plant and helped it to grow fruit,

grains, or vegetables for you to eat. You might wish to say
grace aloud or silently, using words you learned as a child or
making up your own.

Step Six. Eat mindfully. Notice what is on your plate and
your fork, notice how it feels when you put the food in your
mouth, and notice how your whole body feels as you eat.
Pay attention to your hunger signals, and eat slowly and
mindfully.

At-Your-Best Eating

I'm not going to tell you exactly what you may or may not eat. This
is not the typical weight-loss book or program, nor is it meant to provide
you with the latest breakthroughs in magical weight-loss formulas. You
know your body better than anyone else does. And, you might even have
a library filled with diet books, cookbooks, and the like. Yet, if you're
here now with me, I bet you'd agree that knowing it all hasn't helped
you up until now, has it? You have to commit to this program one day at
a time and make it workable for you. Be radically honest with yourself
about what your body needs and what you need. I'm going to set forth a
simple plan for "at-your-best" eating.

My clients and students who have had the best success with the
weight-loss program simply avoided all sugars, most stimulants, and all
processed refined flour. I am happiest and at my best when I do this, too.
I know that if I listen to that noisy food I'll quickly return to disordered
eating. Once I've eaten it, I get cravings and start sailing down the
River of Denial, telling myself that it's okay, I can eat "just one." Who
am I kidding?

Sugary, fatty foods that appeal to our brain's pleasure centers tend
to be noisy, but so do foods made of processed or refined flour. Refined
flour acts on the body like sugar, spiking your blood sugar quickly and
causing blood sugar fluctuations that lead to food cravings. Think of it as
just another form of sugar. It makes sense to avoid any food that triggers
food cravings, especially if it's high in calories, but for some of my clients
who had success with the Weight Loss for People Who Feel Too Much

program, I suspect that removing gluten, a key ingredient in grain-based foods, was important, too. These days, many people have low tolerance for gluten or even have celiac disease, a severe food intolerance, and shouldn't eat even a small amount of it.

Gluten, the protein that makes bread stretchy when you pull it apart, can be found in products made with wheat, rye, and other grains, but if you're gluten intolerant, you might have trouble digesting rice and oats as well. If you can tolerate gluten, make sure your breads, pastas, and cereals are whole grain, meaning they contain the entire grain, including the fiber found in the hull or husk. Your body needs fiber for a healthy digestive system. And don't be fooled by "multigrain" breads that are made with highly processed flours, dyed brown with natural food dyes, and have about as much fiber as a marshmallow. If it's squishy, it's not whole grain!

In addition, in at-your-best eating, you should avoid *all* stimulants and depressants, especially if you know you depend on them to manage your moods and your energy level. If you can't operate without three cups of coffee, or you can't get through the evening without a glass of wine before dinner, you're relying on these foods for mood management and fuel. Don't worry—you're going to learn plenty of healthy techniques for perking yourself up or relaxing. The coffee, caffeinated tea, sugars, colas, and alcoholic drinks won't be so tempting once you've started working with the exercises in the book.

Drink plenty of water to stay hydrated, and try to abstain from processed foods that have been highly altered from their original, using everything from high temperatures to chemical treatments, and which include all sorts of artificial ingredients including artificial flavorings, colors, and preservatives. Processed foods are often packaged and prepared with nitrites (think sausage and luncheon meats), bleached flour (the wheat flour is chemically treated to make it look whiter), refined sugars, and hydrogenated and partially hydrogenated oils (also known as trans fats). If the label has a long list of ingredients, many of which you can't pronounce, or your grandmother would not recognize as food (where exactly are the nuggets on a chicken, anyway?), you probably shouldn't eat it. And if the precooked version of what you're about to eat looks like the pink slime some fast-food restaurants put in their meat products, think long and hard. Should you be eating that? Just saying.

Eat lots of fresh food, and make most of your food plant-based.

If you're not a vegetarian or vegan, and you choose to eat fish, poultry, meat, and dairy, eat cleanly. Avoid processed meats and cheeses, and, as mentioned, buy organic foods whenever possible. You'll learn later why I recommend not eating factory-farmed meat or dairy products at all, but you don't have to be a vegan or vegetarian for this weight-loss plan to work. I have gone through periods of being strict vegetarian, then vegan, and now I feel better eating fish; I will have grass-fed humanely slaughtered beef a couple times a month. It's personal for each of us. For now, just eat simply and concentrate on eating mostly plant-based foods that contain no additives and eating cruelty free.

Go ahead and have some fruit, and if you like fruit juice, drink it in moderation—just a few ounces a day (you can mix it with water) so you don't take in too much sugar at once. Just be honest with yourself; if you are drinking lots of juice because you crave the sugar, cut down or cut it out altogether. I love carrot and beet juice. Of course I do! It has the highest sugar content of any vegetable juice. Be aware of your choices.

Second-Best Eating and Off Days

If you normally use sugar as a sweetener, try to go without. If you can't, use a little maple sugar or syrup, dark agave sugar, stevia, or unprocessed honey (don't use fake sugars like aspartame). Using healthy sugars, eating some processed foods, chowing down on white pasta, and having a latte or a cocktail isn't strictly forbidden, but it is *second-best eating*. You can do better—try to avoid these foods completely. Coffee? Tea? Green Tea is your best option, but if you're like me and love your coffee, buy organic coffee and make it at home; and if you can, make it with alkaline water to cut down on the acid in it (more on that later).

That said, you are going to have off days, when you just have to grab for cookies, chips, candy, cake, or other comfort foods to deal with feeling too much. These are not "Faturdays," as my girlfriend Jennifer calls them: "cheat days" when you plan in advance to eat a piece of chocolate cake for dessert. These are the days when you don't just sneak a latte with a tablespoon or two of sugar, you eat a huge frosted sugar cookie or a candy bar (or two or three) furtively in the bathroom when no one is looking—or you pretend you're sick so you don't have to go out with others, preferring a good old-fashioned binge in the comfort of your own home. *But it doesn't count if no one sees it and I eat over the sink.* Wrong!

On these days, when you recognize you're about to eat a food that's on your "avoid" list, ask yourself, *Is this what I really want right now?* If the answer is *no*, abstain. If the answer is *yes*, go ahead and eat a small portion of that food on a plate or napkin or in a cup or bowl. Do this even if you bought it from the gas station checkout display or a vending machine at work. Having comfort food once in a while isn't bad or wrong—it's how you eat it. A great rule of thumb is this: if you can't eat it in public, right out loud and in front of people, and you only want to eat it when no one's looking, it's not the right choice. That would be a *no*.

To maximize your chances of sticking to at-your-best eating, don't skip meals, be sure you have access to healthy foods when you're likely to be hungry, and eat mindfully. Serve yourself the food, sit for a moment, and either do the Landscape of Your Hunger exercise described earlier in this chapter or go through the steps of "how to eat" before you take a bite. The more off days you have, the more important it is to slow down and work with the exercises in this book, which will help you melt away your resistance to changing your eating habits and will teach you better ways to manage your feelings of being overwhelmed. Practice self-compassion and be radically honest with yourself about what you're eating and why.

In her 1982 book, *Calories Don't Count If You Eat Standing Up*, columnist Barbara Halloran Gibbons introduced the idea that we tend to ignore the excess calories we consume by coming up with absurd excuses for why they don't count. The idea took off and many people have added to it. See if you've been kidding yourself by subscribing to the "dieter's rules" below.

Dieter's Rules (or, The Lies We Tell Ourselves!)

- If you eat while standing over the sink, walking down the street, or driving, the calories don't count.
- If you eat and nobody sees you eating, the calories don't count.
- Broken cookies and candies are calorie-free because all the calories fell out of them when they broke.
- There are no calories in fudge you buy in a gift store while you're on vacation. The same for ice cream eaten while on vacation, or at least with children nearby, and alcoholic drinks consumed at weddings, Bar Mitzvahs, high school reunions, etc.
- Foods eaten in the movie theater contain no calories, so go for the buttered popcorn and "theater size" Junior Mints. In fact, there also aren't any calories in buttered popcorn or theater-size candies as long as you eat them while watching a movie at home or on a portable device.
- A diet soda eaten with candy, cheeseburgers, or cake will render them calorie-free.
- Whatever you eat as comfort food or to self-medicate when you're feeling lousy is calorie free, whether it's frozen custard, cheesecake, cookies, good wine, or cosmopolitans.
- Halloween candy does not contain calories as long as you're eating it to prevent cavities in your children's teeth.
- If you lick the spoon, the knife, or the mixing bowl, good news—no calories!
- Food eaten off children's plates to prevent wasting it has no calories.

Wrong, wrong, WRONG!

How many dieter's rules have you invented to make up for grounding yourself with foods and overeating?

Fortunately, as you learn to better manage your porous boundaries and be mindful of your body's needs, it'll be even easier to stop kidding yourself about the movie Milk Duds and the leftover pizza on your child's plate.

If I'm Eating So Well, Why Do I Feel So Awful?

Some of you may find that when you clean up your diet as part of this weight-loss program, right away you will feel some discomfort: headaches, sluggishness, irritability, and so on. This can happen when your body starts clearing out the toxins that have built up in it. I know—it seems unfair that when you start eating well, you get socked with a stomachache or a migraine, but it's all good. When the toxins are out of your system, you'll feel better than ever—and you'll be more cautious about putting them back into your diet.

Detoxifying can also bring up emotional toxins, like anger, fear, grief, and resentment, that you've buried deep inside you. Drink lots of water, be self-compassionate, and let yourself feel the emotions so that they can dissolve naturally instead of getting stuck inside your energy field and your subconscious mind. Use your journal to express your feelings as you go through this detoxification. And you can tap-tap-tap it, too! *Even though I feel like total crap, I love and approve of myself!*

That's it: kindness, IN-Vizion exercises, salt, and simplicity (simple plans for eating and movement, simple emotional field). They are the four key ingredients for making this program work for you. So, get a hold of the salts and essential oils; make a trip to the store to stock up on healthy, natural foods (mostly plant-based); find two journals, one for the Dumping Grounds and the other for Solutions and Insights; and let's get started with Step One: Speak Your Truth.

KEEP IN MIND . . .

- People who feel too much tend to go back and forth between being very emotional and avoiding emotions altogether. As you learn to manage your emotions and your porous boundaries, these wild fluctuations will decrease. Your emotions will settle down and you won't feel so compelled to ground with food.
- Disordered eating leads to weight gain, eating the wrong kinds of foods, and blood sugar fluctuations that tax our bodies.
- Besides grounding with food or eating in a disordered way, we detour around painful emotions by obsessing over food and weight and setting up unrealistic goals for eating. Working this program will help with this unhealthy eating pattern. Pay attention to any signs that you have an eating disorder and need professional help.
- Avoid noisy foods: those you crave for physical and emotional reasons because of their associations (such as salty processed foods, or the sweet treats you used to make with Grandma).
- While working this program, hide your scale. How your clothes fit is a better indicator of whether you're losing or gaining weight.
- Eat slowly and mindfully. Every meal has to have a beginning, middle, and end. No eating standing up or kidding yourself about calories consumed while you're on the run and avoiding your emotions!
- Every morning, write in your journal what you intend to accomplish. Each evening, write in your journal about how well you did and why, and identify at least one thing you did right.
- Do any daily journal writing required the first week of each step.
- Be kind to yourself. Battling your weight or your body is counterproductive. Be loving and self-compassionate and you'll see better results.
- Use the IN-Vizion Process. IN-Vizion exercises, scattered throughout the book, are great ways to access your hidden,

inner wisdom and process painful emotions using prompts for
visualization.

- Do a Himalayan salt bath ritual daily at 4:00 P.M. (when you
can), incorporating the Emotional Freedom Technique of using
affirmations and tapping to clear up disturbances in your body's
energy field caused by your thoughts or emotions. You will wash
off the emotional garbage of the day and relax as a result. If you
need to, do a saltwater spritz and change an article of clothing at
4:00 P.M. and do the bath later in the day. Use a combination of
pure essential oils, Epsom salts, and the highest-quality Himalayan salt.

- Keep it simple. Follow a simple eating plan, do simple movement, and maintain a simple emotional field. Avoid stimulants
and depressants such as coffee and alcohol and consider cutting
out sugar and gluten, which can be noisy foods that trigger disordered eating. Don't worry about exercise; just move your body
to stay healthy. Avoid stimulating your emotions by consuming
media.

PART THREE

Four Steps to Managing Your Porous Boundaries

Step One: Speak Your Truth ("Yep, I'm a Person Who Feels Too Much!")

You have probably suspected for some time, maybe even most of your life, that you're a little different from other people. You feel more deeply and are more sensitive. You have difficulty separating yourself from other people's emotions. You are powerfully affected by anger, grief, and fear that isn't your own. Somehow, you're just more vulnerable to the emotional energy that surrounds you.

Can you own that? Can you admit to it? Can you say aloud, "Yep, that's me, I'm a person who feels too much!"

Speaking your truth is difficult because it requires that you acknowledge your vulnerability. You have to be honest with yourself and then, eventually, be honest with others, too. That's especially scary because you have to carefully choose the people you'll confide in. I'm asking you to speak your truth to yourself so that one day you can speak your truth to those who are closest to you.

When you're not honest with yourself, when you desperately hide your truth from others out of shame, you inadvertently set yourself up to experience even more misery. You start to think you're doing just fine keeping a lid on your feelings and then *smack*— emotional overload hits you like huge wave, engulfing you. You detour into disordered eating, caregiving for others' emotions, isolating yourself, or other unhealthy behaviors in an attempt to escape that tsunami of emotions.

It's human nature to overestimate how easily we can manage our feelings, our thoughts, and challenging situations. We adopt a "can do" attitude and ignore the little voice whispering, *Actually, I'm not so sure. After all, I've failed before.* What we need to do is hear that voice, hear our doubt, and consciously choose to have faith in our ability to establish new habits through practice.

Our willpower and our capacity for denying the truth about ourselves can be quite strong and impressive. Without realizing it, we put all our trust in the power of our conscious mind and its "can do" attitude, and we rely on willpower to keep us on the path we want to be on. We forget the influence of our *subconscious* mind, that shadowy place where we store the truth; that we've tried again and again to lose weight but failed; that we've tried to manage our anxiety, but it still gets the best of us, that we haven't completely rid ourselves of low self-worth. Deny the truth and it will always surface, usually in a way that makes us very uncomfortable.

Step One in managing your emotional and empathy overload, and in learning to control your porous boundaries, is to speak the truth *unapologetically*, without shame or embarrassment. You've had a problem for as far back as you can remember: you become easily overwhelmed by your emotions, you eat to manage the distress you feel, and you've lost faith in yourself. None of that makes you weak, bad, or inadequate.

Speaking your truth is liberating and empowering. All the energy you've been spending in denying that you're emotionally overwhelmed can now be redirected in a positive way. You can love yourself as you are right now, and at the same time you can eagerly embrace the process of learning to manage your feelings and your porous boundaries.

If you think back to times when others have taken advantage of your vulnerability, of course you're going to feel upset and embarrassed, and you fear that you'll be taken advantage of again. Deep down, you're wondering, *What if I speak my truth and look into the abyss of no solution? What if I'll always be so sensitive, and I'm destined to experience suffering more than others do?* Now there's a series of thoughts that will lead you to obsess about cupcakes.

It's hard to admit to patterns that have caused you pain, but once you do, that marvelous quality of empathy can begin to serve you instead of enslave you. When you speak the truth, as you will on your journal pages, you value your feelings and, by extension, you value yourself. Then, when you've spilled your pain and anguish onto the paper, you can make a conscious choice to hold on to the emotions or to let them go. *You* have the power of choice when you're not operating out of denial and shame.

Some of you have already discovered the incredible tool of journaling: recording your thoughts and feelings in a private notebook. You know that you feel better when you acknowledge what you're experiencing and write your truth. However, if you're like me, you've also gone back to those journals later and thought, *Oh, wow, am I a mess. How depressing. Am I really that screwed up and unhappy? Ouch!*

As I explained in Chapter 3, I want you to journal in two separate books during this program (more during the active weeks than during the processing weeks). I want you to hold on to your beautiful, empowering affirmations and to the insights that give you strength and comfort. Keep those in your Solutions and Insights journal and revisit them. Just be aware that some of what you'll be writing—maybe much or even most of it—will be venting and belongs in your Dumping Grounds journal. Later, you'll reread the Dumping Grounds journals to look for insights and revelations and will write about those in the Solutions and Insights journal.

Journaling is a practice that will get you into the habit of observing yourself. In Step One, you will begin by telling the story of your struggles with empathy and your weight.

YOUR STORY OF EMPATHY AND WEIGHT

One of the most common detours of people who feel too much is isolation. We withdraw from others because intimacy is incredibly intense for us. It's not that we don't love or want to be with others, but that confusion over "Where do I end and you begin?" is scary and makes us feel unsafe. Avoiding people seems like a good option, and it can be at times—sometimes, we just need to be alone—but it's not good to isolate yourself too much. It's far better to have enough control over your porous boundaries; you make a conscious choice about whether you want to pull away from people temporarily or allow yourself to be fully emotionally present with them even though they are angry, sad, or anxious.

Over time, if we isolate too often, we learn to hide our feelings not just from others but even from ourselves. The longer we go on avoiding difficult feelings, the harder it becomes to experience *any* feelings. Instead of avoiding suffering and being happy, we just feel . . . nothing. Being numb is no way to go through life, but neither is being in a constant state of emotional agitation. You have to manage your emotions so you can feel joy, delight, amusement, faith, gratitude, and so on—all the emotions that get stifled when you isolate yourself and cut yourself off from the risk of suffering.

If your story has many painful elements, it may be difficult for you to write it, but it's important to speak your truth. You can't change the past, but you can change the present and the future by choosing to validate and honor yourself for having the strength to survive what you have survived. You don't have to get stuck in the story of your past, playing the role you have always played. Your history should be a guidepost, not a hitching post. In speaking your truth, in writing your story, you free yourself to tell a new one: a story of a person who suffered but learned, and grew, and changed. It is a unique story, but at the same time it has universal elements. When you realize that, you'll find it easier to believe that all around you are people who, if they heard or read your story, would reach out to you with love, compassion, and acceptance.

One of the most powerfully healing aspects of AA is that people share their stories and speak their truth, without varnishing it, and they find acceptance and fellowship. You may not be ready to share your story publicly, and you can choose to keep the details to yourself if you like. However, recognize that if you do reach out to others who have had similar experiences, and to others who simply have a great capacity for compassion and kindness, you will find that you don't feel such a need to isolate and be secretive.

As I said before, all of us have stories that are unique but that have common threads. None of us is alone in having porous boundaries and in experiencing empathy overload. You might be surprised to find out how common your story is, and how many people understand why you are the way you are, and would readily accept you as is, not as "inferior goods." I think we often are so hard on ourselves that we can't imagine other people would have a different opinion of us—one that's much kinder and more loving.

So what is your story? Below are the questions for you to answer in your journal this week. I suggest you answer three or four every night until you've answered them all. Also, be sure to start each morning by journaling your answer to the question, "What is my intention for the day?" and end each night by journaling your answers to these questions:

How did I do?
What is one thing I did well today?
What is one thing I am grateful for?

DAILY JOURNALING FOR STEP ONE:
SPEAK YOUR TRUTH

Write the answers to the following questions in your Solutions and Insights journal (not the Dumping Grounds—save that one for venting later on). Allow at least 20 minutes for this process each day for 7 days, and answer 3 to 4 questions a day.

1. As a child, were you oversensitive? Hypervigilant? Give examples.

2. What does it feel like to have no boundaries?

3. How have you tried to distract yourself from your feelings?

4. As you look back on your life, what was happening the first time you gained weight?

5. What was going on when you lost weight, if you lost it at some point?

6. Have you ever gained or lost weight without changing your food choices?

7. What thoughts have you had about your body?

8. Have you ever tried to control your weight consistently? How long were you able to sustain that sense of control?

9. Do you eat at night? What are your nighttime eating habits?

10. What are your noisy foods, the ones that trigger disordered eating?

11. What happens when you begin to eat a noisy food? What happens after you've consumed it?

12. What would your life be like if you were able to consistently manage your porous boundaries?

13. What would you lose?

14. How would you be different?

15. How do you think others would treat you?

16. How does being someone who feels too much serve you?

17. What does "cheating" on a "diet" do for you?

18. How do you try to manage your empathy?

19. Do your methods for managing empathy work for you? If so, what happens when you use them? Are there long-term effects? And are those positive or negative?

20. When your techniques for managing empathy don't work, what happens?

21. If the coping and self-protection practices you've used were not effective and healthy, can you accept that you need to replace them?

22. If the coping and self-protection practices you've used *were* effective, and healthy, can you accept that you need to use them regularly?

23. What would your life look like if you could love and accept yourself and find a way to reduce the empathy overload that feels overwhelming?

~~~~~~

Take a look at the themes in your story. The participants in my Weight Loss for People Who Feel Too Much class found that they had one or more of the following experiences:

1. They seemed to have been wired since early childhood to be very sensitive and empathetic.
2. They experienced a great loss, such as the death of a parent, brother, or sister in their childhood.
3. They experienced abuse as children and perhaps as adults, too.

Any child who has lost someone close, particularly if it's a parent or sibling, will naturally feel unsafe, as will a child who has been abused. In response, she will become hypervigilant, wary of the next painful experience. She'll become attuned to what others are feeling, to the point where she can pick up on tension as if she had antennae sticking out of her head. She will also have difficulty trusting others and either avoid intimacy or try to achieve it too quickly, extending trust instantly in the hope of securing it and settling her fear. Is this ringing any bells for you?

The stories of people who feel too much also have other themes in common:

1. *Caretaking for others at the expense of yourself.* We all need to help out other people at times, but people who feel too much take on far more than they can handle, to their own detriment. They have trouble saying no to requests for help, and are the first to jump in and offer it.
2. *Standing up to bullies.* Even as young children, people who feel too much were likely to stand up to kids, or even adults, who bullied other children. They can't stand watching someone

suffer and feel they have to get involved. Sometimes, they are more upset by these incidents than are the actual victims of bullying or teasing.

3. *A strong sense of justice.* People who feel too much are keenly sensitive to unfairness. As children, they may refuse to play musical chairs because it just seems so *wrong* that the aggressive kids get chairs and the gentler kids end up losing their seats.

4. *A habit of isolating.* Isolation can take the form of avoiding people or simply avoiding emotions, conflicts, and difficult discussions—whatever it takes to hide from painful feelings!

5. *A tendency to avoid stimulation.* Some people become night owls to avoid the stimulation of busy days filled with people. Others avoid crowds and gatherings, even happy or celebratory ones. Parties and gatherings can be overwhelming because of the influx of emotions and stimulation, or because the person who feels too much wants to make everyone happy and comfortable and is terrified of disappointing anyone.

6. *Difficulty receiving support and guidance.* Not wanting to appear vulnerable, or not feeling deserving of help, or both, often prevents people who feel too much from reaching out for help or accepting support when it's offered.

7. *People pleasing and too much concern about what others think.* People who feel too much spend a lot of energy worrying about how others perceive them and feel about them. They go out of their way to be ultra-nice, always helpful, and super-reliable so that no one will ever be disappointed in them or irritated with them.

8. *Being overly serious or overly comedic.* Because of their anxiety and feelings of being unsafe and vulnerable, people who feel too much can be too serious and have trouble lightening up. They don't want to let down their guard and risk offending anyone or opening themselves up to criticism. On the other extreme, other people who feel too much use humor as a means to deflect the energy of others and protect themselves by being funny.

9. *Having been "10 going on 40" as a child.* Whether they were hyper-responsible and quiet, or bossy and controlling, people

who feel too much often developed behavior patterns in childhood that made them seem older than their years. As adults, they may be overly involved in others' lives, or take responsibility for their parents and adult siblings. They may be helicopter parents, too, constantly fussing over their children and worrying about them. If someone anywhere in their vicinity is upset, they feel it's their job to cheer them up and fix their problems.

10. *Rebelliousness.* Breaking the rules helps a person who feels too much to see where he ends and others begin. At the same time, rebelliousness can upset or anger other people, so the rebellious person who feels too much may feel guilty and ashamed but be unable to stop rebelling, either. Being able to cheat on a diet or secretly sneak in extra calories is one common form of rebellion; acting out sexually, such as being promiscuous or cheating on a partner, is another form. In the moment, it feels good to be rebellious, but then we realize we've sabotaged our goals and we feel ashamed. One of my workshop participants found that as she did the journaling work in Step One, she got into a "frenzy with food," rebelling against the simple plan of eating because of the strong emotions she stirred up. Rebelling against our conscious, healthy choices, resisting new behaviors, is common in Step One and Step Two.

11. *Emotional oversensitivity that was clear even in childhood.* People who feel too much often have childhood memories of being far more sensitive than other kids were, avoiding Three Stooges movies, Road Runner cartoons, and the like because even mock violence was disturbing to them.

12. *A feeling of being the odd one out.* Unaware that others may also have very porous boundaries and are deeply empathetic, people who feel too much often feel like "the odd one out." They perceive that others aren't so sensitive or so prone to taking on others' emotions.

It may seem that some of these themes contradict each other: being rebellious versus a people pleaser, for instance, or isolating versus caretaking for others. You might vacillate between two seemingly opposite behaviors, trying to find balance and become centered, but always, somehow, going to an extreme to manage your emotions. The following quiz can help you start thinking about how empathy overload puts you out of balance, and what it would look like if you could stop being turned upside down and inside out by emotions you take on.

• THE EMOTIONAL MANAGEMENT QUIZ •

1. **When you hear through friends that someone you used to know in high school has been diagnosed with terminal cancer, you:**

A. Feel sad and a bit wistful about the old days, reminisce about how healthy and vibrant this person was in high school, then post a nice note on his social media page or ask your friends to pass along your good wishes.

B. Contact your old friend and offer to help in any way you can, keep checking in with his wife or your mutual friends, and visit him in the hospital. You cry for him and feel grateful for your own health.

C. Find yourself crying on and off for weeks and feel depression overcoming you. You want to visit your old friend but the thought overwhelms you with sadness, and then you feel guilty for not following through on your intention.

D. Become so distraught that you're distracted and depressed or anxious for days, and become so involved in helping him and his family that they seem taken aback by how much you're doing for them, which makes you feel uncomfortable and confused about whether you're doing the right thing.

2. **When someone harshly criticizes you, you:**

A. Have little emotional response, and quickly assess whether that criticism is true and can be used to help you improve yourself in some way.

B. Instantly feel hurt and perhaps angry, but then you walk off your frustration or talk it through with someone and come around to accepting the criticism or rejecting it.

C. Feel devastated, deny to yourself and anyone else that you were hurt or upset, yet stew for days about the incident.

D. Feel furious, confront the person angrily with evidence that his criticism is completely unjustified, and afterward feel a whirlwind of shame, anger, and sadness.

3. **When you find yourself in a large crowd, unable to move as freely as you would like, you:**

A. Consider your options, such as finding a less crowded spot where you can get your bearings. You may feel mildly frustrated with the lack of movement, but you're not bothered by the situation and you easily make your way to a quiet area.

B. Feel somewhat anxious and frustrated, find a less crowded spot, or decide to leave the event or situation. You go home disappointed and a little unsettled by the experience, but you're glad you made the decision to leave an uncomfortable scenario.

C. Feel very anxious and frustrated, even angry or panicked. You find yourself pushing through the crowd aggressively or hurriedly escaping. Afterward, you realize you're breathing shallowly and your heart is pounding, and you want to be completely alone for a long time.

D. Feel overstimulated and unsure of whether you're fearful, irritated, or excited. You're mesmerized by all that's going on around you and start talking quickly to strangers around you, trying to get a handle on what's happening.

4. **Two strangers suddenly get into heated argument in front of you. You:**

A. Keep your distance, watch quietly, and assess whether this may turn violent and whether you should take out your cell phone and call the police.

B. Observe the strangers closely to determine whether you should intervene in some way, and feel your heart pounding and adrenaline pumping. You know better than to get between them physically, but you're carefully eyeing them and trying to decide whether you should say something to try to calm one or both of them.

C. Feel panicked and experience shallow breathing, a quickened heart rate, and a sense that you're in danger. You make a fast getaway but feel upset for hours afterward as you worry about whether you did the right thing.

D. Feel energized and stimulated, even angry, and decide you'd better intervene in this argument right now before someone gets hurt. You immediately become involved without stopping to think about whether it's safe to do so.

5. **You are at a workshop, church service, or other event and you notice several people becoming teary or are quietly crying. You:**

A. Observe their emotional response and think it's appropriate, but are slightly embarrassed by their emotional display. You feel sentimental or sad too, but you don't cry in public.

B. Become teary too, and feel a sense of connection and intimacy with the strangers around you. You share a smile, a hug, or a tissue with someone else and even make a small joke about the strong response you're having.

C. Feel nervous and choke back any tears of your own. You hate to have others see you cry. Uncomfortable, you look for the nearest exit.

D. Feel a sense of excitement at sharing such a powerful experience with others and begin to cry freely. Suddenly, you realize you've unleashed a flood of emotions and you begin sobbing. You're embarrassed but unable to stop yourself because the feelings are so powerful.

6. **Your friend is telling you about an incident at work where a coworker openly ridiculed him and others laughed. He's angry and hurt. You:**

A. Tell him that such a response indicates that his coworkers do not have a healthy working dynamic if that's the way they behave. You start a dialogue with him about how to manage their behavior and whether to approach the supervisor about the chronic problems in the office.

B. Get upset for him but tell him it's his coworkers who have issues, not him. You gently reassure him that any mistakes he made were understandable, and give him a pep talk. Afterward, you feel glad you were able to help your friend

but you're no longer upset; you trust your friend to work
it out.

C. Say nothing as you start to think back to times when you've
been ridiculed. A sense of shame overcomes you and you hold
on to it for hours. You avoid talking to your friend because it's
just too painful to hear his stories.

D. Go into action mode, telling him what to do, and spouting off
about his horrible coworkers. Afterward, you go home and can't
stop thinking about it, and even turn it over in your mind in the
middle of the night. You wake up determined to talk to him
about the incident again.

7. **A friend asked you to commit to helping her with an event and
you quickly agreed, but now, on second thought, you're realizing that it's too much of an imposition and you want to back
out of your commitment. You:**

A. Call her and tell her you spoke too quickly, apologize, and say
you'd like to help but need to make less of a commitment of
time, or take a rain check for a time when you haven't so many
other commitments.

B. Hem and haw about whether to get out of it, and finally make
a decision based on your gut feeling that this just isn't a good
time for you. You call your friend and apologize as you bow
out of the commitment. If you're pressured to reconsider, you
hold firm despite feeling a bit anxious. Then, after hanging
up the phone, you take a deep breath and let any unpleasant
feelings go.

C. Find yourself angry and resentful toward your friend for
pressuring you and to yourself for so quickly agreeing. You
can't find the courage to confront your friend. You don't show
up at the event when you're supposed to. You know your friend
is angry, you feel guilty, and you hole up at home, berating
yourself for how you handled the matter.

D. Start stressing out because you really don't have the time
to help your friend, but you wouldn't dream of backing out
after you said yes. You throw your schedule into turmoil as
you scurry to meet your commitment, and feel guilty about
the appointments you miss. You engage in disordered eating
because you're working crazy hours to get everything done.
Even so, you wouldn't dream of saying anything to your friend
about how stressed out you are.

8. **You turn on the television and see coverage of a terrible earthquake and injured people wailing. You:**

A. Feel sad and sympathetic, then follow the instructions on screen to make an instant donation to disaster relief. You decide to watch the news for a few minutes to get the gist of the story, then turn it off because you feel you've learned what you need to know. After all, suffering is part of the human condition.

B. Feel deep sadness and even begin to cry. You make a donation to disaster relief and spend a few minutes thinking about the victims, even praying for them. Then, feeling a sense of gratitude for your own safety, you turn off the television and hug your spouse, child, or pet. You consider getting involved in disaster relief and make a decision based on whether you can afford to make such a time commitment right now.

C. Become utterly paralyzed with grief and shock. Your eyes become glued to the television and you start surfing between the 24-hour news channels, trying to learn as much as possible because you feel you owe it to the victims to hear about their pain. You don't sleep well or function well for days, and even writing a check to disaster relief does little to help you return to a state of peace.

D. Become deeply upset, then stop everything to become involved in disaster relief. You become obsessed with posting about the disaster on your social media accounts every hour or so, and consider taking a leave of absence from your job to travel there to help, even though you have clients and family dependent on you. You don't have a passport, you haven't any specialized skills for helping, and yet you can't let go of the idea that *you* have to travel to the disaster zone to help out.

9. **You are visiting a memorial to a tragic event, and find yourself in the building where people suffered terribly years ago. You:**

A. Soberly reflect on the suffering, perhaps say a prayer, and leave, having been moved by the experience.

B. Feel yourself deeply moved and tearful. You say a prayer, make a deeper commitment to your own efforts to help the world in your own way, and vow to visit memorials like this more often in order to connect with the importance of the work you do to serve humanity, however humble that work may be.

C. Become nauseated and short of breath, and have to run out of the building. You don't regain your equilibrium for a long time, and vow not to go to any more such memorial sites in the future.

D. Find that tears are streaming down your face. You ask the guide to tell you more about the suffering of the people involved, and how you can get involved in supporting the memorial and the causes it promotes. You can't stop talking about the experience for weeks, and start to obsess about it.

10. People who know you well would describe you as:

A. Very logical and rational.

B. Compassionate and levelheaded.

C. Extremely sensitive, moody, and inconsistently intimate with people.

D. Highly emotional and dramatic, always involved in others' emotional dramas.

11. When it comes to people and pets who need help, you:

A. Are sympathetic but let people solve their own problems; you write checks to your favorite charities and perhaps do some volunteer charity work that you find rewarding and fulfilling.

B. Are sympathetic and even empathetic, truly feeling their distress, their joy, and their anxiety. However, you have your feelings and moods under control so that you're able to serve others without becoming drained. You know how to pace and replenish yourself.

C. You become overwhelmed by the suffering of others and, much as you'd like to help, you're too distraught to reach out to people; instead, you tend to reach out to food to ground yourself.

D. You are quickly sucked into the emotional experiences of others and become angry or zealous as you try to solve the problems of the world. You try to ground yourself with food when you start becoming overwhelmed, but it's so hard for you to slow down and rest that you often become physically or emotionally burned out.

Scoring

Mostly As: *Logical Thinker.* You rely more on logic than emotions to make decisions, and your thoughts dominate your feelings most of the time. This causes you to be sympathetic but not empathetic: you feel for others but you don't feel, or take on, their pain or strong emotions.

Mostly Bs. *Balanced Feeler.* When you make decisions, you rely equally on logic and emotions. You're able to be empathetic and truly feel other people's strong emotions, but have strong boundaries that allow you to remain grounded and centered most of the time.

Mostly Cs: *Isolating Feeler.* Your emotions dominate your decision making and can be quite intense. You're very empathetic, and you respond to taking on others' strong emotions by withdrawing and isolating yourself.

Mostly Ds: *Connected Feeler.* Your emotions dominate your decision making and can be quite intense. You're very empathetic, and you respond to taking on others' strong emotions by trying to become closer to them, either through caretaking or by getting drawn into the drama as a player who hopes to direct the action and make the situation better for all involved.

How balanced are your feelings? Can you imagine being able to feel emotions without having them knock you over and cause you to isolate or become too involved in other people's problems?

You may have learned growing up that love means always being connected, even if it's painful. Have you met people who take the attitude, "If you really love me, you'll engage in a drama with me?" Do you have close family members and friends like that? It's hard to set healthy boundaries with people you love if this was the message that was drilled into you in your youth!

In my home, my mother didn't let me close my bedroom door and would walk into the bathroom anytime she pleased, regardless of what was going on in there. It wasn't intentionally intrusive, but boundaries just weren't allowed in my house. Survivors of sexual abuse and rape have a very difficult time setting healthy boundaries, too. My mother and I were both victims of sexual violence, and I believe those experiences contributed to the unhealthy survival skills we both exhibited around intimacy. Consequently, I've had to learn to establish new patterns in this area that still can cause me to pause before I remember it's okay to take care of myself.

Don't forget that you can always visit the inner sanctuary you created and experience safety, and there, you can even meet your childhood self and reassure and comfort her.

SOURCES OF SHAME

Too often, people who feel too much have shame that goes all the way back to childhood. It seems to me that shame is a very destructive feeling because you can't do anything with it—you can only feel bad. Anger, fear, jealousy, or embarrassment can wake you up to something you have to address, but shame puts you into a state of inertia. It cripples you when what you need is self-love, strength, and optimism to help you make changes. It makes you identify with your negative behaviors, so that you don't see yourself as a good person who has taken some actions you're not proud of; you see yourself as a bad person who will always be bad and will always take actions that feed and perpetuate your shame. The deep embarrassment that we are not whole, that we hide a terrible secret that will inevitably prove us to be unlovable, unworthy, and a living mistake, is reinforced by our own desire to disown the part of us we think we need to hide.

We people who feel too much have lots of shame about eating because our eating patterns are tied up with our emotional patterns, and we're ashamed of our inability to control our empathy overload and porous boundaries when it seems everyone else can do it. We compare ourselves to others and think there's something wrong with us, that we're somehow damaged. We eat to ground ourselves and carry great shame about that, so we hide the eating. At the same time, many of us—particularly those who grew up in a household where we developed a fear of scarcity—hide what we're eating in order to be sure that no one takes our food away from us. This is a very emotional behavior and we can be very irrational about our secret stash of caramels or potato chips. In fact, children who have experienced emotional trauma very often will steal food and may hide it rather than eat it, just to reassure themselves that they are in control of the food, that they will never be without. Sneaking food can feel like an assertion of the self when we're feeling the discomfort of being flooded by feelings that aren't our own, when we feel our porous boundaries are wide open and taking in all the emotional energy around us.

We also will often be secretive about the amount of food we consume. We'll snack before going out to lunch with friends so we can pick at a salad and pretend we really don't eat all that much. We eat the fine chocolates, remove the empty wrappers from the box, and carefully rearrange them to make it look as if the box is still full.

What messages about shame and control have you internalized? Think about the source of those messages. For instance, did you have an overweight mother who was terrified that you, too, would be overweight someday, stuck in an unhappy marriage, and unable to attract someone else? Did your mother control the amount and type of food you ate, and use treats to reward you? Were you jealous of one of your siblings, and did you respond to your feelings of being not good enough by secretly bingeing? Did you always dream of having the "good snacks" your wealthier cousins or playmates had, and associate name-brand goodies with being safe and secure?

Maybe there are identity issues around what you eat. Some children are ashamed of the foods at their families' tables—too ethnic, too fancy, too cheap or plain. Did you grow up longing to eat certain foods in order to be like everyone else? Eating is a very social event, and as social creatures, we want to fit in.

I remember how ashamed I was when I was a girl and my mother insisted on giving me coarse rye bread with salami and cheese for lunch that had a distinct European smell, as opposed to the peanut butter and jelly my friends were eating. My decidedly Canadian friends in my grade 2 class made fun of its odor and moved to another table, which really hurt. I can also remember how my mother made a beautiful German al-mond cake and brought it to our annual bake sale at our school. No one bought a slice of her cake because it wasn't "Canadian." She was upset when she brought it home uneaten, and I felt the shame of how different we were from the others. It was in the early 1960s and I imagine World War II was still fresh for some people, so German food seemed somehow suspicious to them. Although I have come to accept and love that I come from a different ethnic background, those memories still sting.

Maybe as an adult, you find your family and friends tease you when you eat differently from how they do. If so, how does that make you feel? Are you taking on someone else's attitudes about eating and weight? Have you internalized them? Most important, are you ready to let go of those attitudes that are holding you back?

A LONGING FOR SAFETY

By now, you realize that feeling safe and secure is very important to people who feel too much. It's hard to control that anxious response to empathy overload or strong emotions. In fact, you feel it so intensely it's actually a strong physical sensation. Learning to make peace with the more difficult emotions is crucial to the success of this program. Know-ing that "this too shall pass" and approaching your experience in small increments, maybe even one hour at a time, makes following the pro-gram so much easier. People who feel too much tend to feel assaulted and invaded by the energy of the world, which leads to isolation and/or other detour habits to avoid uncomfortable emotions. This sense of thin or porous boundaries makes for a tremendous amount of distress and discombobulation combined with worry and anxiety.

Again, while some people just seem to be born highly empathic, a great number of people who feel too much are affected by something in their past that caused them to become hypervigilant and hyper-intuitive. They may have had their boundaries trampled owing to being sexually abused or raised in families where there was an absent parent, fighting and rage in the home, or alcoholism or addiction. It's not difficult to see the genesis of the "I'm not safe" message for people who grew up in these types of environments.

Food is the gooey, crunchy, salty, sweet, all-encompassing, yummy safety blanket, the escape, the momentary inhalation that brings relief from the lack of safety. Weight acts like a wall between you and the world, preventing intimacy, attempting to create a force field that serves as a boundary.

Bessie is a woman from Texas who called me for a session a few years ago, before I decided to put this program together. When she and I spoke on the phone for the first time, she told me she wanted my help in figuring out why her marriage was unraveling. Yet, the conversation quickly moved to discussing her history with weight issues. She kept gaining weight, and didn't understand why she couldn't stop eating. Bessie felt there was nothing she could do about it. On top of that, she was convinced her husband was having an affair, since they'd had little or no sexual contact since the birth of her second child, who was now an active 5-year-old. Having dieted since she was 18, Bessie, now 42, weighed 300 pounds. She told me there had been a few times when she had lost a substantial amount of weight, but then as soon as she was close to her goal, she would start experiencing anxiety and gain it all back.

I brought the conversation back to her emotional situation, and Bessie confessed that her husband was an angry man and that she could feel it coming off him like "steam off the griddle." I asked her how she felt about her husband and her eating. "Horrible," she said. "He calls me a 'heifer' and other names."

I just wanted to jump through the phone lines and hug Bessie because I could totally relate. I'd had a similar experience with a man I dated in my early 20s who would taunt me whenever I gained a few pounds, and would refer to me as "Little Lotta" after a chubby, dark-haired, pigtailed character in kids' comic books.

Bessie, like many others and me, had spent most of her life riddled with fear and shame, anger and self-reproach. When we began to speak about her childhood, she told me she had always felt too much, and she sensed the anger in the air in her family's house, especially when her father would come home after a long day's work. Her father, a store manager, drank his way through dinner, then plunked himself down in front of the TV until she went to bed. He was gruff and distant, and would often fly off the handle at her mother, which of course, scared Bessie.

She remembered that she always had some kind of candy stash, which she would eat whenever the emotional temperature in the house got too heated. Her weight steadily grew into her adolescence when the yo-yo dieting began. It was worse when she went to college, although she recalled having a couple of years at a time where her weight melted off her as she increased her dieting resolve. Then she would fall in love and as soon as she got close to the man, her dress size would go up. The fear of becoming too close to a partner wasn't conscious, but it drove her to disordered eating and, inevitably, she would gain weight. She laughed when she told me she had a wardrobe in enough sizes to start her own clothing store. In her Southern drawl, she said, "Hell, you know, I just want to feel safe inside my own skin and I know cupcakes aren't the answer!"

Like Bessie, many of us find that food makes us feel safe, then robs us of the very security we think it can offer us. We lose our sense of power over our choices, then revert to using food as comfort and protection. Then the weight piles on and the self-worth goes down.

Feeling safe in your own skin is important. Feeling that you have the power to set boundaries, and not be swallowed up in intimate situations, and to make healthy choices is tantamount to healthy self-esteem. It's important to know that safety is a state of mind. You can learn how to feel secure and practice feeling that way until it becomes second nature.

As you work this program, you'll find yourself feeling unsafe less often, and the insecurity that arises in you won't be quite so intense. Remember, whenever you feel threatened or insecure, you can use the IN-Vizion Process that you learned earlier—the Discover Your Inner Sanctuary exercise—to create a sense of safety.

THE TRUTH ABOUT YOUR DISORDERED EATING

One of the truths you must speak is the truth about your disordered eating. Take this Disordered Eating Quiz and see if you can identify your disordered eating patterns.

• THE DISORDERED EATING QUIZ •

1. **When your schedule is changed suddenly because of an unexpected event you have to attend, you:**

   A. Come up with a plan for picking up a healthy meal on the go and healthy protein snacks to tide you over to the next meal.

   B. Decide you'll just grab the healthiest food you can when you get really, really hungry. You figure you can eat better and according to schedule tomorrow, yet somehow you always seem to have a poor diet.

   C. Worry about whether you'll have enough to eat, and head to your pantry and fridge to wolf down what you can just in case you get stuck with no access to food—then end up snacking mindlessly throughout the event.

   D. Convince yourself that everything will be fine, start to feel very panicky when you get hungry, and end up eating half a pizza and a decadent dessert afterward because, after all that stress, you deserve it. When you finish eating, you feel ashamed.

2. **Your usual eating pattern is:**

   A. Three meals and two healthy snacks a day.

   B. A healthy, light breakfast to start, then somewhere around midday, the plan for healthy eating goes away, so that by the end of the night you're not sure what you ate or when.

   C. A rigid plan for three low-calorie meals and no snacking, which never seems to work out because you actually eat all day long but rarely have a square meal.

   D. You either have no eating pattern or an extremely rigid one that isn't healthful and which you have strong emotions about.

3. **You wake up in the middle of the night and scrounge for a snack:**

A. Never.

B. Rarely, but you do snack throughout the day, "grazing" or nibbling here and there, but you've read that's a healthy way to eat. Still, your weight and mood are not what they should be and you have to admit, your "grazing" foods include more cookies and white bread than raw vegetable sticks.

C. Sometimes, when you're under a lot of stress. The bigger problem is that you have vowed never to snack but find yourself doing so regularly, and snacking on junk.

D. Almost always. You can't help it.

4. **It's holiday time again, and you've scheduled several parties where there will be calorie-laden holiday foods. You:**

A. Come up with a reasonable plan for what you'll consume and stick to it for the most part.

B. Come up with a reasonable plan for what you'll consume, then discover afterward that you gained several pounds in a week.

C. Vow not to eat any holiday goodies at all—then find yourself bingeing on treats at the very first party you attend.

D. Figure, "What the hell? It's the holidays," and tell yourself the weight gain won't be significant.

5. **When it comes to vegetables, you:**

A. Eat five to eight servings a day of them daily, usually steamed, raw, or sautéed.

B. Intend to eat them, but find it easier to grab a sandwich because you always seem to be famished and on the go with no time to prepare meals.

C. Have dozens of recipes and cookbooks with vegetable-based recipes in your kitchen, but you're constantly throwing out spoiled produce, and mostly you eat vegetables in the form of french fries.

D. Gave up on vegetables long ago, although you do eat fruit here and there.

6. To you, the perfect meal would be:

A. Balanced in color, nutrition, and texture, served at the usual time, and enjoyed with friends or while sitting in a beautiful spot.

B. Delicious, filling, healthful, and inclusive of a rich dessert, but very low calorie and available at any food court or minimart when you're on the go.

C. Prepared by someone else because you haven't a clue what constitutes a healthy and delicious meal.

D. Anything involving yummy food, food, food!

7. When it comes to weight loss and gain, you:

A. Have mild fluctuations in your weight but can almost always attribute these changes to differences in how you're eating or how much exercise you're getting.

B. Experience big weight swings that seem to have little to do with how much you're eating or exercising.

C. Set out to lose lots of weight, get frustrated by your progress, binge, and watch your weight balloon, much to your dismay.

D. Are waiting for the magic pill or operation that will fix your weight problem once and for all so you don't have to think about it because you've tried everything and nothing works.

8. The noisy food that seems to call out to you "Eat me! Eat me!" is:

A. Nonexistent. You don't have strong cravings for foods and you eat a balanced diet that includes the occasional sweet treat, junk food, or rich entrée.

B. Chocolate—no, wait, chocolate cake—no, potato chips. The sour cream and onion ones. . . . Well, anyway, there are some noisy foods.

C. Nonexistent. You don't have strong cravings for foods and you eat a balanced diet that includes the very occasional sweet treat, junk food, or rich entrée. That bag of mini candy bars in your desk drawer and the huge chocolate chip cookie you buy when you get your 3:00 coffee every workday don't count.

D. Just about everything in the junk food aisle or the deli counter at the grocery store, so you dread going grocery shopping because it's all too tempting.

9. Maintaining your weight is:

A. Fairly easy.

B. Impossible; in fact, you're not sure what the right weight for you should be.

C. An endless battle for you and you never seem to win.

D. Something you try not to think about. It's easier to simply wear loose clothing and not own a scale.

10. When it comes to how the people who bring your food to the table and the animals that become your food are treated, your attitude is:

A. Eat organically, close to the earth, in a sustainable and humane way.

B. I wish I ate better, and I hate to think about what they do to those cows and chickens on corporate farms, but it stresses me out to think about the origins of my food because I feel so little control over what I eat and how it got to my plate.

C. Eat organically and cruelty free at all times even if you have to go without. You are a rigid vegan and are horrified by people who eat hamburgers. You've been known to lecture people about what they eat.

D. Whenever I look at food, I feel guilty because I can't stop thinking about the poor cows and chickens, the underpaid migrant workers and grocery stock clerks, and those who go without food. The only thing that helps me feel less upset is to eat, eat, eat, but then I feel ashamed afterward.

Scoring:

Mostly As: You probably don't have disordered eating except in rare circumstances, but you might want to gather a few more helpful ideas about eating and weight maintenance.

Mostly Bs: You may be in denial about how disordered your eating is. This book will awaken you to how much your "eat on the go" habits are affecting your weight, mood, and health, and how much your emotions are affecting your food choices.

Mostly Cs: Your eating is disordered because you anxiously set unrealistic goals and, understandably, fail to achieve them. This book will help you let go of your guilt, shame, and anxiety and help you start creating some realistic goals about food and weight that are rooted in a healthy sense of self.

Mostly Ds: Your eating is disordered because you have no food and weight-loss or weight-maintenance goals. You simply go for the gusto when you see food and feel awful afterward. This book will help you get to the root of why food and weight are such issues for you.

As you commit to giving up disordered eating and instead eating mindfully according to a simple plan, you're bound to be a little resistant. How does it feel to control your eating and have a beginning, middle, and end to every snack or meal? Are you worrying too much about what you're eating and when, and using perfectionism about eating as a detour?

Some of you may go back and forth between bingeing and deprivation, or even bingeing and purging: you binge when you're on empathy or emotional overload, and you purge or start to restrict yourself when your feelings simmer down and you suddenly become aware of your rising shame and guilt. You want to self-correct—and you overcorrect. It is very important that you allow yourself off days and that you develop a new habit of responding to any binges by exploring your emotions and processing them. Feeling ashamed blocks you from that exploration. Look at that binge or that off day as an opportunity to make some serious progress in empathy management. Aim for progress, not perfection. As soon as you notice you've engaged in disordered eating, stop what you're doing, find a quiet place, and do the following From Here to Your Sanctuary exercise. (If you didn't do the earlier exercises on creating an inner sanctuary and identifying your food landscape, do those first, as this one combines them.)

FROM HERE TO YOUR SANCTUARY

Whenever you're feeling agitated by any strong emotion, close your eyes and take a few deep, slow breaths, concentrating on your breathing. Ignore any thoughts or word messages that come up and let your subconscious mind speak to you through pictures.

Continue to breathe in and out, slowly. Hold on to one intention: seeing a landscape that reflects what you're feeling at this moment. Ask yourself,

Where am I?

Allow your imagination to deliver the answer. It always will, by the way. Observe the landscape or place that appears before you. If it's not very detailed, that's okay. Simply observe it and its features. What's the weather like in this landscape? Is it storming? Gloomy? Windy? Notice the state of the sky and the ground beneath you. Are the skies threatening? Is the ground secure beneath your feet?

Even if you are scared, remain here long enough to take in the details of the landscape, then look into the distance, toward your sanctuary.

Does it feel far away?

How do you feel now looking at the place?

Connect to the sensation of being the observer of it, rather than the person feeling the emotions. What is blocking you from getting to your sanctuary? Are there any obstacles in your way?

Now notice something in the landscape that will take you to

your sanctuary. It may be a giant bird that swoops down and picks you up, or a bridge, or other means for escaping to the landscape you'd like to be in.

Remember that this is *your* place, *your* imagination, and you have the power to summon anything to reach the Sanctuary.

Now, take your escape. Then savor the feeling of being in your sanctuary.

When you are ready, open your eyes and think back to the first landscape. What did the features of that land represent? How did you interact with the land? What does that tell you about where you were emotionally a few minutes ago?

How did you escape the land? What does that tell you about your power to shift your emotions? What landscape did you find yourself in?

You may find it helpful to describe the exercise in your journal. Don't analyze it until you have written down all the details you remember about the landscape, your sanctuary, and how you got from the distressing landscape to your sanctuary. Then you can let your logical mind figure out what the symbols mean.

Later, you will explore this landscape more, when you've gotten more practice at using the IN-Vizion Process and tolerating difficult emotions. For now, know that even though you might end up in that distressing landscape again, at least now you know how to escape it and get to your sanctuary.

~~~~~~

When you feel on the verge of eating a food that's noisy for you, you can use the From Here to Your Sanctuary exercise and then ask yourself, *Is this what I'm hungry for?* You might be surprised by how much easier it is to walk away from that noisy food when you use this simple process before putting the food in your mouth. Remember to write in your journal to speak your truth about your experiences and feelings, because this will help you to develop the habit of managing your porous boundaries and difficult, powerful emotions. On off days, it's especially important to speak your truth as you write in your journal pages.

As you become more mindful of your noisy foods and the emotions that make foods noisy for you, you may realize your disordered eating is more problematic than you thought it was. Some of you might sense that you have the symptoms of an eating disorder. Denial is a huge part of eating disorders, and that confused, distorted thinking is easier to correct when you get the nutrition your body and your brain need. If you even suspect you have an eating disorder, or your friends and family are worried about you, please read about the symptoms, below.

SYMPTOMS OF ANOREXIA NERVOSA

People with anorexia nervosa obsess over foods and thinness, and they starve themselves. Symptoms include:

- very low calorie intake
- skipping meals
- a distorted body image and self-image (do your friends say you're too thin or that you're not eating enough?)
- ritualized eating of a very limited number of foods (for instance, only eating parts of lettuce leaves)
- using medications and supplements for weight loss
- dry skin, hair, and nails
- hair loss and loss of muscle tone
- bones sticking out because you're so thin
- soft hair recently appeared on your body
- loss of menstrual period, or irregular period
- fear of gaining weight or eating too much
- stomach pain or bloating
- mouth sores
- feeling cold most or all of the time, low body temperature

- tiredness
- low blood pressure
- ignoring hunger signals to the point that they may even disappear
- dehydration, thirsty all the time
- constipation
- extreme exercising
- defensiveness about your weight and eating
- lying about what you eat or weigh to keep others from criticizing you
- isolating in order to avoid uncomfortable questions about your eating and weight
- disguising your thinness with baggy clothing

SYMPTOMS OF BULIMIA

Bulimia involves bingeing on large quantities of food (typically, a noisy food for you), then causing vomiting afterward in order to rid yourself of the calories. Bulimics may be thin, overweight, or in between.

- eating a large amount of calories very quickly
- eating so much, so quickly, that you feel physical discomfort
- feeling disgusted and ashamed after eating a large amount of food
- fear of gaining weight, which doesn't prevent the bingeing
- constantly thinking about food, eating, dieting, and exercise
- eating alone or privately, fear of eating around others, sneaking food
- irregular menstrual cycles
- dry skin, hair, and nails
- hair loss or muscle tone loss
- mouth sores

- stomach pain or bloating, gastrointestinal problems such as acid reflux and gas
- dehydration
- tiredness
- erosion of tooth enamel from vomiting
- sore throat, inflamed salivary glands

If you feel obsessed about dieting, eating, weight, and your body, or you have symptoms of an eating disorder, you may have one of these life-threatening conditions. Seek help. *Listen to the people who care about you if they express concerns.* They can help you.

Compulsive eating is a maladaptive way of addressing a very real underlying problem of empathy overload. If you find yourself obsessing over food or experiencing depression and anxiety, you might have a nutritional deficit you don't know about that, once addressed, will balance your body's biochemistry and change your mood and thoughts (more on this later in the book—for now, pay attention to what are your noisy foods).

HANDLING EMOTIONS

Speaking your truth also means letting your emotions surface and acknowledging them. This is difficult for people who feel too much, because we become so overwhelmed by emotion that we can't sort out what we're feeling. It's as if our emotions were one big ball of pain. Some of my workshop participants realized they were avoiding the 4:00 P.M. bath because they knew that, once they stepped into the tub, the emotions would flow and they'd feel scared and ungrounded.

Here's the secret about emotions: they don't last. When you actually let them surface and don't try to justify them by creating all sorts of thoughts that perpetuate them, they peter out fairly quickly. It doesn't feel that way when they come up suddenly and they're intense—it seems that you'll feel like crap until the end of eternity! However, if you make sure you are in a safe place, alone, when you get in touch with your feelings, they will rise and fall naturally in a matter of minutes. Often, our emotions surface at very inconvenient times, and we're so afraid of being out of control that we learn to stifle them—and do, every time.

Of course, you don't want to burst into tears when you're talking to your boss, or cut loose your anger when you're talking to someone you care about, but once you're alone, do you stop to let your feelings surface? Probably not. The moment has passed and you move on, but your emotions remain stuck inside you. Then, if you stay busy enough, and repress your strong emotions every time you feel them start to bubble up, you can maintain that false sense of control for quite some time, maybe even years. Maybe you always run late because you fear that if you have a few minutes' downtime, awful memories or feelings might emerge. Avoiding emotions doesn't make them go away, though. It just means you end up spending enormous amounts of energy trying to keep a lid on them.

When you learn to let your emotions rise and fall, in a natural rhythm, you'll find that they aren't as strong and difficult to manage when they come up unexpectedly in conversations with others or situations where you'd be uncomfortable expressing them.

Emotions will rise when you're in the bath and as you write in your daily journal. Let them, and just observe them. Breathe deeply while you're experiencing them. Ask yourself, *What is this emotion?* Don't think about *why* you're feeling it until the emotion has passed. That way, you won't accidentally intensify it through negative self-talk.

Another way to bring up the emotions you need to feel and let go of is using *cinematherapy*. Choose movies to watch that you know will make you cry or get you in touch with your anger. Try to watch them alone so you feel safer when your emotions surface. Afterward, take out your journal and write about what you felt and why. Finally, ask yourself, *Did*

I see myself or others in those characters and those situations? In fact, if you see a movie just for fun but it really upsets or unsettles you, and you don't know why, take the time to get your journal out and write about what you just experienced.

I think it's an especially good idea to watch movies that will make you cry but have uplifting endings that leave you with a sense of hope, joy, and optimism. For example, you might watch *The Joy Luck Club*, *Water for Elephants*, *It's a Wonderful Life*, or *Ghost*. Keep the tissue box handy and don't let your partner, your kids, or anyone else interfere with your good cry!

What if the emotions you're feeling actually belong to someone else or to the great ether—what if they're something you picked up from the electromagnetic field we all share? Cinematherapy and the IN-Vizion exercises are effective ways to let go of them. Then, to help ground yourself when you're feeling empathy overload, you can try the following two exercises as well: The Slick Blue Shield and Them's Grounding Words.

THE SLICK BLUE SHIELD

Close your eyes and breathe deeply and consciously. Let your thoughts float away like clouds in the sky. Allow yourself to feel your emotions without thinking about them or justifying them.

Now imagine that you are surrounded by an egg-shaped, brilliant blue-neon bubble. The surface is oily. All the emotions and thoughts that come at you from outside of you hit the surface and slide down like raindrops dripping down a window. You are safe inside this bubble. Even if you are feeling strong emotions, they are going to dissipate soon. Continue to breathe.

Observe yourself as a sense of calm and safety fills you.

Open your eyes when you are ready.

THEM'S GROUNDING WORDS

One of the easiest ways to ground yourself when you feel caught up in a ball of confusing emotions and are outside of your body is to say your name, the date, and your location, and name the objects around you: the chair, the kitchen table, the phone, the sink, and so on. Actually speak the words aloud. When you do this, you will feel yourself coming back into your body and bringing your rational mind back online. My certified Weight Release Energetix coaches work with clients using a process called Counting, which on its own is like the above description or is used as a component of the IN-Vizion Process when someone gets stuck inside his or her own imagery. It's highly effective and actually a lot of fun to do.

I have heard from many of my course participants that getting out in nature, even for just a short walk, helps them to ground. Also, you might find that if you push together or pull apart your joints, an action that provides something called *proprioceptive input,* and get deep pressure against your skin somewhere, it can help you to feel present in your body again. Think walking, jumping, pushing or pulling something, calisthenics, hugs, and massages. This is called "heavy work" by occupational therapists who work with people who have sensory-processing issues (they process physical sensations atypically). These therapists often suggest that people who have sensory issues do heavy work throughout the day to prevent that overstimulated, overwhelmed feeling. In fact, many people who feel too much also experience sensations more intensely, and they may have sensory-processing differences (more on this later in the book in the section on movement in Chapter 7).

THE TRUTH ABOUT SELF-TALK

If you don't believe in the power of positive affirmations and self-talk, guess what? Even the U.S. Navy SEALs have discovered the effectiveness of actively replacing negative self-talk with positive affirmations. When we change our internal chatter to have a positive quality, our primitive, limbic brain, which is responsible for setting off a fear response of fight or flight, begins to calm down. The power of positive thinking is even stronger if we're also using a visualization or doing something physical to quiet our system. In moments of stress, there's actually more blood flow to your limbic brain, and less blood flow to your prefrontal cortex where you can think clearly, make good decisions, and check your impulses. Saying to yourself *I'm okay. I can handle this* really does help you think clearly and feel more balanced.

Remember: words create emotions, and emotions have a biochemical reality in our bodies. When you replace your negative interior dialogue with positive thoughts, the cells in your body respond. With practice (and, yes, you have to practice!), you can replace that endless disempowering chatter with a positive string of beliefs—and you will believe *I am beautiful, I love my body,* and *I deeply and completely love and accept myself.* These become your truths. Make sure your self-talk nurtures and supports you.

What sort of things are you telling yourself regularly that you're not mindful of? What's the quality of your self-talk? Pay attention. Are you harshly judging yourself as fat, crazy, or inadequate? Create affirmations that are in the present tense, and make sure they're positive, not negative; for instance, *I love my body,* not *I don't hate my body.* If you find yourself resisting the affirmation, reword it. You have to believe what you're saying and feel positive emotions for affirmations to work.

Using positive affirmations is part of the EFT ritual you'll be using daily in your salt baths, although, as I pointed out, you construct these particular affirmations by combining the difficult truth about what's going on with you ("Even though I ate a huge piece of pie . . . ") with a positive statement ("I deeply and completely love and accept myself"). It is very important to speak your truth! In your journal, write down some affirmations and memorize them—and find times throughout the day to repeat them silently or aloud. The EFT only takes a minute or two to do, so you can start creating a habit of doing it a few times a day. In this way, you'll retrain your inner dialogue track.

That said, it's okay to laugh at yourself and use humor to bring yourself back into a positive state. One woman I know responds to frustrating and disappointing situations by saying, "Well, now, this is *exactly* what I wanted." It's such a huge lie that she can't help laughing. Everyone has a different sense of humor. If there's a funny mantra that will make you smile, or even laugh out loud, and will shift you out of anger, frustration, or sadness, use it!

As you learn to speak your truth, you're going to feel more powerful and much safer. You'll realize that the earth isn't going to shift beneath you and the sky isn't going to come crashing down just because you are finally being honest with yourself. The new techniques you're using will bolster your ability to speak fearlessly about where you are in your life and in your process of learning to manage your porous boundaries.

PROCESSING IT ALL

When you begin to sort out your emotions and recognize the many different threads that together are the fabric of your life, you start to recognize your truth. The process of uncovering and speaking your truth takes time. Be good to yourself, and be patient. You may need to devote more than a week to doing the journaling exercises in this chapter so as to deeply explore what your story and your truth are. There's no one standing over you saying you must complete this step in exactly two weeks. Only you can judge how much time you need before you're emotionally ready to move on to Step Two.

All processes take time. In fact, think about processed foods: they're meant to be time savers, right? Crack an egg, beat it, and add it with some oil to a cake mix and you're cooking from scratch—well, not quite.

Some clever businessperson figured out many years ago that you could fool homemakers into thinking they were baking it, not faking it, by leaving a few ingredients out of the cake mix. Do you do that in your own life? Do you take shortcuts in your process of working through your emotions? When you do, you don't get the results you want.

Because you are taking on others' emotions, and so many of them, you might require more time to process your feelings than other people do. You may need lots of downtime with a journal, in nature, or meditating to get in touch with that tangle of emotions and process them. Life is so fast-paced these days that it's hard to take a breath before you are hit with a new piece of information to digest, or a new emotional experience to make sense of.

In this weight-loss program, there are no shortcuts. Speaking your truth ends the detour of denial and saves you a lot of time and energy. You get straight to the issues you need to deal with and avoid the detours that take you far off your path. This is difficult work. If you decide you need more than two weeks to work through Step One, be sure to do your daily journaling exercises during week one, writing your story, then follow through with the daily baths, the simple eating plan, morning and evening journaling, and journaling whenever you're moved to do so or you've done one of the exercises and want to process what you experienced.

When you are ready, and no sooner, move on to Step Two.

Step One, Week One: Exercises and Activities

- Be kind to yourself. (Remember KISS: kindness, IN-Vizion, salt, simplicity).
- IN-Vizion exercises as needed to help you manage your empathy overload and strong emotions.
- Morning journaling: what's your intention for today?
- 4:00 P. M. salt bath (or salt spritz, followed by a bath as soon as you can do it), during which you do the IN-Vizion

exercises and use the EFT and affirmations to speak your truth and process your feelings.

- Follow the simple plan of eating and movement. Continue to avoid physical stimulants and mental ones (such as the news and social media).
- Daily journaling. Answer three or four questions a day, and record any thoughts, feelings, or insights that feel important to you.
- Do each of the exercises within the chapter.
- Evening journaling: How did you do today? What is one thing you did right? What is one thing you're grateful for?

Step One, Week Two: Maintenance
Exercises and Activities

Note that you'll do these basic activities throughout this program and into the future.

- Be kind to yourself. (Remember KISS: kindness, IN-Vizion, salt, simplicity).
- IN-Vizion exercises as needed to help you manage your empathy overload and strong emotions.
- Morning journaling: what's your intention for today?
- 4:00 P.M. salt bath (or salt spritz, followed by a bath as soon as you can do it), along with EFT to process your feelings.
- Follow the simple plan of eating and movement. Continue to avoid physical stimulants and mental ones (such as the news and social media).
- Journal daily or every few days if you find journaling helps you to sort out your feelings.
- Evening journaling: How did you do today? What is one thing you did right? What is one thing you're grateful for?

KEEP IN MIND . . .

- Speaking your truth to yourself is extremely important, which is why journaling is a part of this program even after you finish actively working the four steps.
- Be honest with yourself about your eating patterns and emotions, such as shame and fear.
- Practice self-compassion.
- Getting overly involved in other people's situations in order to quiet your emotional turbulence and avoiding any and every emotion are just two of the ways people who feel too much try to manage their empathy overload. Two more are disordered eating and grounding yourself with food. This program will help you avoid these and other detours.
- Whenever you feel overwhelmed, use the From Here to Your Sanctuary exercise in this chapter to identify your feelings and use your imagination to experience them, then escape to an inner sanctuary. You can also use The Slick Blue Shield and Them's Grounding Words exercises, get out in nature, and do physical movements ("heavy work") you find calming and grounding.
- Be aware of the signs of anorexia nervosa and bulimia. If the people who care about you are worried that you have or are developing these disorders, please seek medical attention.
- Replace your negative self-talk with positive self-talk. Catch yourself being cruel to yourself and stop! Then affirm something wonderful about yourself.

Step Two: Own Your Truth ("Can't I Just Promise to Eat Better?")

So, how are you doing? In Step One, doing the exercises and following the simple plan probably stirred up a lot of emotions for you. At the beginning of any new program for change, it's easy to be brimming over with enthusiasm and determination. Then we all know what happens. We start to realize, *Oh, wow, this is HARD!*

If you're like most people who feel too much, you're used to detouring away from your emotions or being completely engulfed by them, and now you've got more emotions going on inside you than ever before. You're realizing you really do have to end the free-eating habit permanently. It's normal at this point to feel resistance.

Resistance is uncomfortable, but it's good: it's a sign that you're breaking through to something new. In the springtime, seedlings have to push through the hard shell of a seed to germinate, and through the pressure of soil lying on top of them, to reach the sun. It is the only way to reach their potential as flowers, grasses, and trees. Resistance is a sign of progress.

Resistance is also a sign that you have to pay attention to something you're used to ignoring: your emotional reality. Your feelings arise as a result of your conscious thoughts and your subconscious, instant reactions to events. Using affirmations, especially as part of EFT, allows you to acknowledge your self-sabotaging thoughts and replace them with deep self-compassion, which helps you change the patterns of your conscious thoughts.

Your subconscious thought processes are more difficult to manage because you're not aware of them. Also, your feelings move faster than your conscious thoughts do as a result of your brain's very efficient way of processing information indicating danger—well, at least, it was efficient thousands of years ago when human beings were regularly in physical danger. Now that system is overreactive, so that you'll have the same emotional reaction to your partner saying, "Are you sure you really want to have such a big piece of pie?" that you would have if you were being charged by a wild rhinoceros. In time, as you use the mindful techniques in this book, you'll slow down that too-quick emotional response. Then, a thought such as, *He's not trying to hurt my feelings with that question, he's just trying to support me in my commitment to eating healthfully* will have time to form in your brain before the tears of rage and shame well up in your eyes.

My husband is an expert now at entering into the "should you be eating that . . ." war zone jungle with great agility. I will admit that I have, in the past, turned into a raving version of the possessed little girl in *The Exorcist* when he has—or let me rephrase that, when I *perceive* that he has—crossed the line and entered sacred territory as I am stuffing myself with a second helping of popcorn. He doesn't mean to be the food police, but I have been known to go into spasms of rage when he dares say a word about my moving to Snackville. These skirmishes are rare now, mostly because I don't really overdo it. That said, we have had a recent run-in that makes for a good story.

Toward the end of writing this book, I developed a medical condition. I was having an ultrasound to check out a knot I'd discovered in my neck, when it was discovered that I had a large nodule on my thyroid. Now, I've taken thyroid medication for years for an underactive thyroid, and lately I'd been feeling cold a lot, had some memory problems, and been tired and wired, but I hadn't put it all together. I have been working out three times a week, and I didn't realize that I had some minor inflammation and water retention as a result. In short, I have definitely been having a challenging time with my weight, and I am aware that on a daily basis I have to practice self-compassion with a little more fervor than normal. I am normally comfortable in my size 8/10 skin, but not so much with the widening of the waistline that's been happening for months, partly due to menopause, partly due to my thyroid. The doctor said the presence of the nodule indicated I would have to change my medication, which led to a little more weight gain, which sent me into a tailspin of true paranoia and nightmares of having this book come out and being thrown off *The Today Show* because I was fat. (I actually had a dream that I was set to go on a book tour, but when I arrived the room was silent and then all the press started shooting pictures that landed on the tabloids saying, "Fat Girl Fraudulently Pens Weight-Loss Book and Loses Everything.")

One would consider that would be enough impetus for super-clean eating and wonderful, consistent self-acceptance. If you believe that, then pigs have wings. After being told it would take around three months to get my thyroid issues under control, I somehow "decided" that my two cups of air-popped popcorn was just not going to be enough as my snack. (Carved into the temple at Delphi, it says "Know Thyself," so since I do, and since I am by nature a glutton, measuring for me is a safety mechanism; I know that two cups is enough for me.) Marc watched me get up from the couch and head back into the kitchen to refill my bowl, which I convinced myself had shrunk in the dishwasher. He said in his very blunt Aries way, "Don't you have any willpower? Are you allowed to have a second helping?"

Now, for a moment I felt that rhino charging me across the savannah, and I went quickly over the edge to find my weapons. But before I opened my mouth for a sharp retort and crazy spear shaking, I was able to breathe and ask myself what I was hungry for and what I was trying to escape. I recognized that I was afraid, and that Marc was trying to support me. I managed to put the bowl down and return to the couch, where he sat all tensed up preparing for a fight; but when I squeezed his hand and said, "Thanks, honey," he relaxed into the safety of the couch and managed a deep sigh. It was surrender—not just willpower—that got me to put the extra popcorn back in the bag. I surrendered to the truth that I am a person who feels too much, who detours through disordered eating, and I chose to love myself enough to do what I needed to do for myself at that moment. Denial of my feelings leads to powerlessness, and by now I know that no amount of food will relieve the anxiety; it will just make it worse.

I haven't always surrendered to the truth. I was overwhelmed by emotion after I'd lost my mother in a short period of time. I decided I just had to go out and buy cakes for people to consume after the memorial service. The more I thought about it, the more I needed to get them. I went to the bakery and felt jittery and agitated, and when the baker behind the counter asked what I wanted, it was as if my mouth had been hijacked by the Cookie Monster. I began lying to him about how I was having a party, and would two frosted layer cakes be enough for twelve hungry people, or would three be better? I feared there wouldn't be enough food, a primitive fear I'd inherited from the mother I had just lost. This fear kidnapped my psyche. He said two cakes would be enough, which made me upset; but too frantic and weirdly paranoid to insist on cake number three, I took the two cakes home and ate a huge piece of each one, freaked out, then threw the rest away after mushing them together and dumping pepper and salt on them so I wouldn't fish them out of the garbage. (No one said I was normal.)

Now, I started this manic episode feeling sure that I could control my cravings for those cakes. I had willpower, after all. I would inhale the scent of the bakery, imagine the taste of those cakes in my mouth, and be able to calmly and rationally place my order, take my goodies home, and keep them in the fridge until the appointed time. Uh, huh.

Willpower has its limits. It doesn't reach into your subconscious mind, where you have many self-sabotaging thoughts that cause strong resistance to change. At this point in the program, though, I hope that if you find yourself ripping open a bag of chips while feeling agitated, you're able to stop, catch your breath, and ask yourself, *Wait a minute. What's going on with me? What am I feeling right now? Is this what I'm hungry for?* Cravings can and do have a biological reality, and you can reduce them by cutting out gluten (or at least, refined flour) and alcohol, and limiting your sugars (you'll learn more about the physical basis of cravings later on). You can also reduce the cravings by avoiding highly processed foods with artificial flavorings, additives, and flavor enhancers known as excitotoxins such as MSG, which is sometimes disguised as hydrolyzed vegetable protein, aspartame, or Nutrasweet. These flavorings seem to train the palate to crave more of those tastes because they powerfully affect the brain's pleasure center. However, cravings can also be mostly emotional. Let's face it: few of us have strong positive feelings for, say, lettuce. We associate parties, celebrations, holidays, and special times with sugary, fatty, carbohydrate-laden foods.

Recognize that there are practical ways to ease the intensity of emotional overload, that sense of not knowing where you end and someone else begins. Then you'll have more strength to resist temptation—more than you would have with mere willpower alone—because it's your out-of-control emotions that are driving the disordered eating. Calm the emotional storm, and the junk food won't be so noisy.

Because we feel emotions more intensely than others do, we people who feel too much need to regularly turn inward and experience a place of inner sanctuary. We're not used to doing this, so it may feel uncomfortable, or seem unnecessary, to check in with your inner emotional landscape before you eat—but it is necessary. Perceiving any emotion as a landscape allows you to feel that emotion without being completely caught up in it. This puts you in the seat of the observer: the very important yet rarely accessed part of your consciousness remains aware of your power to notice your emotions and, consequently, learn what they might have to teach you. No learning, growth, or progress happens when you're so caught up in your emotions and freaking out.

And what about the food? If you're frustrated by having to stick to new habits of mindful eating, and with wrestling the strong emotions that keep popping up inside you, that's okay! This is exactly what you should be experiencing at this point, so don't be hard on yourself. Your frustration and resistance will melt away into acceptance if you own the truth of what a huge shift you're making and the challenge of making it. Then it becomes easier and easier to shift your state of mind.

You may be used to pretending you have your emotions under control, and that you can change a few eating habits, or sign up for a diet program that will result in permanent weight loss. However, if you've read this far and have worked Step One, you're ready to own the truth about yourself: you have a chronic problem with managing empathy overload and you respond with disordered eating. And there is no quick fix. You may have to instill new eating habits that take time, even as you're learning to manage your porous boundaries.

Now, you don't have to keep clinging to the lie that you can operate the way you always have and still lose weight, as long as you avoid the cookies at least some of the time. Accept that "watching your weight" and vowing to stay away from sweets or fried foods were never going to make a big difference in your ability to lose weight and keep it off. This situation is way more complicated than that, but there is a solution and you're discovering it here!

THE PROCESS OF GRIEVING AND ACCEPTANCE

Acceptance involves a loss and a grieving process. The late psychologist Elisabeth Kübler-Ross identified the stages of loss as denial, anger, bargaining, sadness, and acceptance. Resistance is what temporarily stops your progress and sends you backward into denial, or square one. When you don't resist your resistance, you remain in the process (which is certainly better than slipping backward into denial!). Resistance makes you uncomfortable and nudges you to practice ruthless self-honesty. It makes you face what you're feeling. Maybe you need to admit that you require more time to work through your anger and resentment about your situation, or your sadness about having to let go of the illusion of control, and your frustration over not being able to manage your emotions perfectly.

Letting go of the lie that we can continue as we always have, only making a few tweaks to our eating habits, isn't easy. Because we tend to be confused by emotions—What are they? Whom do they belong to?—the grieving process isn't always so clear-cut for us. We can vacillate between sad and angry, sad and angry, taking an indirect or circuitous route toward acceptance.

The bargaining part of the process of grieving takes a few different forms. You may try to talk yourself into tweaking the program to get around the most difficult parts of it. Are you avoiding the salt bath because you know that the emotions that flow while you're sitting there will be intensely painful? Are you avoiding the evening writing because it's hard for you to admit that you do anything right without being overwhelmed by sadness that you've spent a lifetime feeling no one notices you unless you screw up? If you're trying to bargain with the program in order to avoid your emotions, you may need some more time with Step One. Reread the exercises about managing your emotions and bringing in positive thoughts using the EFT and the IN-Vizion Process, and do them. (Did you skip them? That's okay—maybe you were scared of churning up strong emotions. Go back and do them now.)

Bargaining also takes the form of talking yourself into stopping the program altogether. You know that's not a logical choice but an emotional one. What you're learning is a new way of asserting yourself and your needs in a way that is not self-sabotaging but, rather, self-nurturing. It's going to be difficult to change your old habits because it will seem more comfortable to go back to the reliable ways of avoiding difficult emotions. It can also be hard to trust yourself to develop new habits when you've failed in the past. It might seem easier to just dump this book and try a restricted-calorie diet again. Skepticism and distrust are typical forms of resistance to doing the work of feeling your emotions, accepting yourself, and committing to a new way of meeting your need for control over your porous boundaries.

If you're ready to give up, again, go back to Step One and work with those techniques a little longer. If you've spent a lifetime keeping a lid on your feelings because they seem big and scary, you may need extra time to slowly move forward into Step Two.

Bargaining can also happen in the moment when you're tempted by a noisy food. You tell yourself that you really are choosing the chocolate consciously even though a little voice inside you is saying, *Hello? Hello? I really don't want to eat this—are you listening? I want you to stop!* You're so overwhelmed by the need to rebel and resist that you silence that voice, saying to yourself, *I don't care what I committed to! I need relief now.* You don't think about the consequences because your need for relief is too intense.

One of the participants in my Weight Loss for People Who Feel Too Much class asked, "How can I not be crazy and fat?" I had to laugh, because that is the central question, blunt though it may be. How can we stop the disordered eating and not be discombobulated by our emotions? How can we manage our emotions and resist the call of our noisy foods that pack on the pounds? We can do it by letting go of the denial that we don't have a lifelong problem with empathy overload and disordered eating. We can do it by surrendering to the roller-coaster process of angry, sad, angry, sad, bargain, sad, angry, bargain, and so on. Own the truth that you're in a difficult process and that you're being courageous in letting go of your resistance.

Finding a reason to give up on yourself and the program is a form of resistance. If you give up, try again. Let go of yesterday. Pick up where you left off.

GOOD-BYE TO SADNESS

In owning the truth that you can't go back to your old ways of distorted eating and out-of-control empathy overload, you have to acknowledge your losses. You're losing food as your tool for self-nurturing. You're letting go of the image of yourself as someone who can avoid pain. You're letting go of the false belief that you are very much in control, and that you're someone who can say, "Screw it!" and eat the cake because she deserves to have it, and then not suffer any consequences for making that choice. Who wants to let go of that belief?

Yes, it's sad that you can't have what you want, when you want it, without paying the consequence. It's sad that you can't easily control your emotions, your empathy, and your response to your noisy foods, as some people seem to. On the other hand, being trapped in the cycle of emotional overload, bingeing, self-loathing, self-denial, emotional overload, and so on is much sadder. The sadness, like the anger and resentment, will dissipate like a big chunk of ice that slowly melts away a little more each time you bring it into the light of self-awareness and self-acceptance. Feeling sadness or anger is painful, but it's soft pain. Hard pain is what you experience when you overeat or when you beat yourself up, and it's much worse than soft pain.

It's easier to accept all these losses I've described and own your truth when you discover new sources of support and new ways to become more self-compassionate. In Step Two, it's important to develop three new habits: to make a point of experiencing joy, to become appreciative of your body, and to awaken your sense of being loved and cared for by a power greater than yourself.

NEW HABIT #1: SAY HELLO TO JOY

Beethoven's Ninth Symphony includes the "Ode to Joy," but we don't exactly sing joy's praises ourselves. In fact, we tend to devalue joy as something that's nice but elusive, and certainly nothing to put much thought into. Doesn't joy auto-load in our lives when we do everything right? Not exactly! When we're happy, wow, do we appreciate feeling joy. When we're sad or feeling challenged, joy isn't on our radar. We forget that we're capable of feeling it. After a while, it starts to feel as if joy is something we have no control over, as if our situations are responsible for our inner feelings. Nothing could be further from the truth.

If you're like many people, you develop "joy amnesia" until you experience it accidentally and think, *Hey, I forgot how good this feels!* How often have you found yourself laughing and smiling, and thinking, *I should do this more often.* Yes, you *should*, but you don't, do you? It's amazing how often we people who feel too much, who are trying too hard to be good people and care for others, forget to experience happiness. Commit to feeling joy more often! There's a whole field of psychology called *positive psychology* that's focused on helping people to identify what makes them feel happy and do whatever it is that leads them to happiness. It seems obvious—do what makes you feel good—but we get a lot of messages about containing our happiness, not being *too* happy or happy too much of the time. We've internalized messages like, "If I'm too happy, I'm tempting fate and something awful will happen," or "If I'm too happy, other people will feel jealous, so I should be careful not to express my happiness," or "If I'm happy, it's because I'm selfish and not working hard enough, because life is difficult and painful." All sorts of ridiculous ideas end up in our heads, sabotaging our joy. Being joyful is our birthright.

What makes you feel energized and happy? Bring it on! Indulge in a funny or romantic movie; watch videos of your favorite pop songs from your youth on social media; hang out on the porch with some old friends, laughing about the absurdities of life. Play a game that makes you feel silly, like a kid. Spend some time around children who encourage you to lighten up and be goofy. Wade into a lake with your jeans on—no one's going to yell at you for getting them dirty and wet now, because you're an adult and you own a washing machine! Seriously, how much do we all hold back from doing something fun because we've got some inner voice saying, *Ooo, that's irresponsible, don't do it!*?

Be spontaneous and adventurous. Pull your car over when you see a county fair and buy a ticket for the spinning ride that makes you dizzy. If you always wanted to take a salsa dancing class, call a friend and ask him to join you, then laugh together if you find yourselves completely inept compared to the so-called beginners surrounding you.

When I turned 53, I got my motorcycle license and now I ride a stunning Softail Deluxe Harley Davidson motorcycle. Although it scared the pants off me in the beginning, I get so much joy feeling the wind against my body and riding along the winding back roads and down the main road by the sea coast where I live. I feel joy in the accomplishment and joy in the freedom it gives me! And I don't care how goofy I look. I make a point to smile when I ride, too.

Do you like to play a musical instrument? If you think you're not very good at it, so what? Play it anyway. No one's judging you. Sing—in the shower, in the laundry room, in the car. Sing out of tune. Who cares? Dance. Draw. Garden. If you don't know what activities make it easy for you to feel joyous, think about it (one of the journal questions in this step is about identifying these activities). Maybe you simply haven't tried enough fun activities to find one that really brings out happiness in you. Try something new. Tag along with someone else to an activity they enjoy. If you don't like it, congratulate yourself for stepping out, and keep looking for activities that make you happy.

People who are positive and who laugh a lot make it easier to connect you to your joy. Make a point of spending time with them. Your environment can make a difference, too. Spend time in a place that fills your senses with delight, whether it's an art museum, a horticultural center, or a gorgeous room with a view of a lake or ocean. Paint the room where you spend the most time a color that invigorates or soothes you. And try the following exercise, which will help you be more aware of how you can adjust your physical environment and make it easier to feel not just comfortable in your space but also happy and even joyous.

CREATING AN EXTERNAL SANCTUARY
OR HAPPY SPACE

When you create an inner sanctuary using the IN-Vizion Process, and visit it often, you'll find it easier to shift out of sadness, anger, or fear and into happiness and peacefulness. However, don't underestimate the power of creating an external "happy space" where you live or work. You don't have to redecorate your entire home, but become aware of your surroundings and how they make you feel, then put forth the effort to make your space more conducive for experiencing joy.

People who feel too much can be exquisitely sensitive to the emotional charge an object or space holds. Are you surrounded by a cacophony of stories encapsulated in your stuff? Do you own furniture that belonged to someone you didn't particularly like or you had a troubled relationship with, and you're afraid to let it go because "it's worth some money" or "it would be stupid to buy something new, so I should get over myself and my feelings"? If every time you look at that object you inwardly wince, stop being practical and replace it. If your closet is full of clothes that whisper to you, "What's wrong with you? Why don't you wear me like you used to? Because you don't have an important job position anymore, nyeah, nyeah, nyeah," shut them up. Get them out of your space.

Once you've eliminated the possessions that wear you down, make you sad, or cause you to be irritable, bring in the possessions that make you feel good, that carry a positive emotional charge. A friend of mine keeps her childhood dolls in her office because they remind her of her rich imagination as a little girl, and they bring her back to the joyful times she spent playing with them. She's in her fifties and couldn't care less if a visitor thinks she's strange having dolls around her desk. It makes her happy.

Put up photos from your cruise or a girlfriend's weekend, use your grandmother's letter opener every day so you can remember back to the magical times you spent at her house playing at her desk—in short, recognize the value of surrounding yourself with reminders of what makes you happy.

NEW HABIT #2: EXPRESS GRATITUDE TOWARD YOUR BODY

The battle against your beautiful, healthy body ends here. Call a truce! Even if your body isn't everything you want it to be, even if your health isn't perfect, your body is well enough to serve you in many ways. Love your body as it is right now and be grateful to it. Although your true identity is as a spiritual being, your body allows you to experience joy here on earth. Affirm *I am strong and healthy. I am only attracted to food that's good for me, that nourishes my wonderful body. Everything that I am resonates health and well-being.* Try doing this while you walk because it will help you to be aware of your body's strength as you put one sturdy foot in front of another.

It's especially important to love the parts of you that you don't want to accept. Here's an exercise for loving your body that you can do before a meal to help you appreciate your body exactly as it is right now.

LISTENING TO YOUR BODY

Before a meal, take several deep, slow breaths. Focus on your body and what it feels like to inhabit it. Feel its strength.

Imagine that your body has a voice. What does it sound like?

Do different parts of your body sound differently or the same?

What other impressions are you aware of? Ask your body,

What do you need?

If you discover that any part of your body is in discomfort or pain, ask that part of your body to speak to you. Ask this part of your body,

How are you serving me?

What gift do you have for me?

What do you need from me?

Listen to the answers.

How are you feeling? Are you hungry right now?

If you feel you want to change the food that is on your plate before you, do so. Then sit down again.

Thank your body for sharing its wisdom with you.

NEW HABIT #3: NURTURE A RELATIONSHIP WITH YOUR HIGHER POWER

A third habit that will help you with acceptance, or in owning your truth, is opening up to support from what I call Spirit, or a higher power.

I know some of you are very resistant to thinking about God, Spirit, or a higher power because you've been treated badly by others in the name of religion, or have seen others hurt by people who call themselves religious. I totally understand that resistance. Or maybe you're fine with it, and Jesus is your savior and your weight-release partner.

But when I talk about Spirit or a higher power, I'm not talking about religious beliefs or theology. I'm talking about creating and fostering a relationship with a loving, supportive force that offers respite from the constant pressures of life. This force is collaborative, providing wisdom, guidance, and energy to help you create the life you long for. It is compassionate and loves you unconditionally. It provides for you in many ways, although it may not seem that way because our vision of what we need isn't as complex and sophisticated as it would be if we could view the fabric of our lives from an eagle's point of view, which Spirit can do.

I have a friend who was angry at God because she developed an autoimmune disorder. She felt it was unfair because she thought of herself as a good person who was always sacrificing for others. Then, as time went on, she came to realize that the autoimmune disorder awakened in her a greater awareness of how she was not nurturing herself and how she could help others to awaken to their need to be self-loving. She realized that, given the path she was on, she might never have experienced the deep personal growth she did and begun working as a healer, if it had not been for the "gift" of an autoimmune disorder. That is, the challenges of her disease were outweighed by her sense of purpose. Back when her doctor first gave her the diagnosis, she had no idea that something good would come out of the bad news he was giving her.

Some of you may feel more comfortable referring to Spirit as God the Father, or He. Don't let me stop you! I just prefer to emphasize the female aspects of the divine force: the qualities of being nurturing, creative, and collaborative. When we connect with Spirit, we experience maternal love and unconditional acceptance, the gentle encouragement to discover our own solutions and create the lives we want with the help of Spirit instead of feeling powerless in the face of fate or destiny. If you grew up thinking that the only way to get God's attention was to admit to how powerless and lowly you are, that belief system can stand in the way of self-love and self-compassion. As you've learned, it's incredibly hard to follow through on your commitment to nurture and love your body when you're feeling terrible about yourself. It's hard to let go of the illusion of power you get when you isolate from others, fight the world by being rebellious, or try to micromanage it through perfectionism—unless you tap into your true power: the power to collaborate with Spirit.

Detours are habits we form to alleviate the discomfort of feeling separated from the divine force, or feeling overwhelmed by empathy overload. We take detours because we think we can find something—some substance, some action, some powerful tool—that will let us fill the great, gaping, Spirit-shaped hole inside us where we yearn for support, love, and acceptance. When we feel connected to the divine intelligence that infuses all creation, the desire for detours starts to disappear along with our habits of isolation, perfectionism, and disordered eating. We are *spiritually* sated because we are nurturing a relationship with the higher power that exists both inside us and outside us.

You are a child of this loving energy. You don't have to solve all problems on your own. When you feel alone and weak, Spirit is there and will send messages to remind you of its presence. What a relief from the constant pressures of life!

So how do we work with Spirit? Some great practices for this are meditation, spending time in nature, and praying.

MEDITATION

There are many types of meditation and they all work well to quiet the chatterbox in your mind and help you feel more relaxed and, therefore, more open to hearing your inner voice of wisdom, which comes from Spirit. Meditation also helps with depression and anxiety. In fact, research led by Sara Lazar, Ph.D., showed that *mindfulness meditation,* which is very easy to do, actually changes your brain, thickening the regions associated with calmness, memory, your sense of who you are, and empathy. Now, I know you're thinking, "Wait, I have *too much* empathy already!" Well, mindfulness meditation strengthens us by giving us a greater sense of clarity and calmness surrounding that empathy, so that instead of feeling overloaded, we experience empathy in a gentler way.

Mindfulness meditation also decreases the thickness of the amygdala, the part of the brain that is responsible for anxiety and depression. It may be that this practice even grows the part of your brain that helps you stay focused and manage your emotions. You can actually retrain your brain in eight weeks using mindfulness meditation for just under a half an hour a day. You can't beat that!

So what does this have to do with Spirit? Well, one of the regions of the brain that is changed by mindfulness meditation is called the temporal-parietal junction, the part where we experience a sense of ourselves as separate physical beings, but also the part that is active when we're having an out-of-body experience, where we feel we're not connected to our separate, physical self. According to neuroscientist Andrew Newberg, in his book *Principles of Neurotheology*, this may be the part of the brain that allows us to feel we are one with the divine, inseparable. Personally, I think becoming more aware of ourselves leads to our understanding that we are spiritual beings connected to a higher power.

Now, mindfulness meditation is very simple to do. Sit comfortably, in a chair with good lumbar support if you like, and rest your hands in a comfortable position. Close your eyes, and as you inhale and exhale, focus on the sensation of your breathing, thinking, "in" or "cleanse" as you inhale and "out" or "release" as you exhale. If thoughts come into your mind or you start to focus on a sensation or something you hear, just bring your attention back to your breathing. Continue for 15 to 30 minutes. That's it!

I like to do mindfulness meditation while listening to a high-quality recording of music designed to alter my brain waves to match certain frequencies known to produce a deep meditative state. Look for binaural recordings (Hemi-Sync Metamusic from The Monroe Institute is one brand I recommend; see Recommended Reading and References). I especially enjoy using one that incorporates ocean sounds. You can also find many of these recordings on my website, www.colettebaronreid.com/weightloss.

SPENDING TIME IN NATURE

Like meditation, spending time in nature has a natural calming effect, but it seems to connect us to our spirituality and to Spirit, too. Frederick Law Olmsted, a Victorian landscaper who designed New York City's Central Park, wrote, "A man's eyes cannot be as much occupied as they are in large cities by artificial things . . . without a harmful effect, first on his mental and nervous system and ultimately on his entire constitutional organization," while time spent in nature is able "to refresh and delight the eye and through the eye, the mind and the spirit." Botanist George Washington Carver once said, "I love to think of nature as having unlimited broadcasting stations, through which God speaks to us every day, every hour and every moment of our lives, if we will only tune in and remain so."

I think part of the reason nature has this effect on us is that we are part of it. When we're outdoors, we're in our home. We experience our part in the vastness of nature even as we're aware that we have the power to crush a tiny violet in the grass or transfer an ant from a leaf to the ground; and we feel that the all is in the small and the small is in the all. Our sense of time shifts as we attune to nature's cycles and observe the movement of the sun and the clouds, the budding of the trees, and the return of birds from their wintering grounds. We feel awe at the creation we get to experience and our humble part in it.

PRAYER

There are many ways to pray, all of which allow us to become used to having a dialogue with Spirit. Saying a supplicant's prayer to our higher power reminds us that we can always count on something larger than we are to help us, and that we're not alone. When we ask for Spirit's will to be done *through* us, we acknowledge that we aren't the only ones in charge of our lives, and we can surrender to the force that provides the underlying order and harmony of the universe. We choose to trust that Spirit has wisdom beyond ours and will share it with us if we still our minds.

When you give your troubles to Spirit, you acknowledge that, as one person, you can't solve everything. What's awe-inspiring is that as you start to practice "giving it up to the divine," you also start to notice that many of your problems work themselves out without your having to devote your mental and emotional energy to solving them. Things just have a way of getting resolved by Spirit. That's why I recommend using a Sacred Box, as described below, to let go of your worries and let Spirit take them over.

THE SACRED BOX

Find a small box, big enough to hold small pieces of paper on which you will have written a sentence or a few words. This space is now your Sacred Box, a sort of mailbox where you can place your troubles, knowing that you're sending them off to Spirit so that you can receive the help and support you need to handle specific feelings and situations.

Any time you feel you can't cope or don't understand what's going on in your life and how it's going to lead to your greater good, write a note about it and place the note in the Sacred Box. If you start obsessing about something, place a description of it in the box. You can place your anger there, or your resentment or jealous thoughts, too. If you're feeling overwhelmed, place a note about it here, being mindful that you are surrendering this to the care of a higher power. Doing this is an act of faith ritualized by having created this receptacle for grace to enter your life. Every six months, or at the end of every year, I take out all the notes I wrote, all the concerns I handed over to my Sacred Box, and sure enough, everything has been taken care of by a force greater than myself.

The Sacred Box probably works so well because making a ritual of a commitment or intention seems to solidify it in ourselves. Although it may seem easier just to say, "Spirit, please take this burden from me," the Sacred Box can be a powerful tool for letting go of worries, too.

LETTING GO OF PERFECTIONISM AND EMBRACING YOUR TRUE POWER

One of the reasons we worry so much is that we can't stand the feeling of being out of control of our porous boundaries and being in empathy overload. Another is that, because we've been heavy, we've experienced judgment and disrespect, even contempt and abuse. Of course, we want to try to take care of every detail so no one can criticize us: *If I'm the good girl, the perfect daughter, maybe Dad won't make a crack about my weight. If I'm an utterly devoted girlfriend, maybe he'll be so attracted to me that he won't notice I gained weight again, or tell me I'm getting fat.*

Are you a perfectionist? Is your anxiety getting the better of you, causing you to try to micromanage the world around you so as to create a stronger sense of safety and control? Take the following quiz and find out.

• THE PERFECTIONIST QUIZ •

1. **You're trying on a new outfit to wear to a wedding or other special event. As soon as you put it on in the dressing room, you:**

A. Glance at yourself in the mirror for all of two seconds, mutter, "Yeah, that'll do," then hurry out to the cash register so you can ring up your purchase and head over to the food court to buy a treat to quiet your anxiety.

B. Take your time looking at yourself in a three-way mirror from all angles, account for the lousy dressing-room lighting that would make any clothing look horrible even on a supermodel, then make a decision based on whether you feel comfortable and attractive in this outfit.

C. Try on the outfit, notice that it might be just a bit tight, hesitate to ask another shopper what she thinks because she might hurt your feelings, and decide instead to ask the sales clerk because you know she'll tell you how great you look. You buy the outfit and carefully file the receipt because you suspect you will exchange it for another two days from now.

D. Try on the outfit and several others several times, then blow your budget buying two or three of them, and vow to skip lunch every day until the special event so you will look good in all of them and can make a last-minute decision.

2. **In your school days, your attitude toward writing a paper or doing a big homework project was:**

A. Wait until the last minute, then try to talk your friend into letting you see what she'd written, and if that failed, you'd wait until the last minute and scribble out something, anything, to fill up the page.

B. Manage your time well so that if you hit a roadblock, you could check with your teacher and feel confident as you went back to working on the project.

C. Rewrite and rework the project again and again up until the last minute, when you ran out of time altogether and had to rush the final steps.

D. Drove your teachers, parents, and friends crazy with your obsessive worrying about how you would do, and ended up crying over minor details at 3:00 A.M. the night before the project was due.

3. **When you discover you've made an error that will affect someone else, you:**

A. Hide it and lie if confronted.

B. Consider how best to break the news and what to offer that person by way of apology, and promptly approach him.

C. Feel guilty, stuff your feelings and binge, and fret about how you'll ever come clean with the other person.

D. Lie awake at night imagining over and over again how you will apologize, and exactly how the person will react, then launch into an inner diatribe about what an idiot you were. You vow never to make that mistake again, *ever!*

4. **Your boss or a client gives you some negative feedback about your work, although in a friendly way. You:**

A. Make excuses and find someone or something to blame.

B. Thank him for sharing, promise that you'll do better next time, offer to make up for not doing satisfactory work, and, without drama, take a few minutes to analyze what happened and how you can prevent it from happening again in the future.

C. Apologize profusely, swear up and down that it will never happen again, and make such a big deal about it that the person feels uncomfortable.

D. Apologize profusely, vow solemnly never to let it happen again, then go home and curl into a ball as you burst into tears.

5. **You just realized you have mindlessly binged on ice cream from your freezer and have eaten half the carton. You:**

A. Quickly put the food away, and tell yourself, "That was no big deal, really," but pick up more ice cream the next time you're grocery shopping.

B. Stop yourself and use one of the techniques in this book, or another you've used successfully before, to get in touch with your feelings and the real reason you're bingeing. You throw out the rest of the ice cream and gently remind your partner not to buy it and leave it in the freezer again. You recommit to working this program.

C. You write six pages in your journal venting about your life-long problem with bingeing on ice cream, then realize you're obsessing just a little too much and use one of the techniques in this book to smooth out your emotional waters.

D. Quickly pull out a calculator, eyeball the portion size you just consumed, read the label, and calculate how many jumping jacks you have to do to burn off the extra calories.

6. **When it comes to cleaning your home, you:**

A. Invest in low-wattage lightbulbs so no one can spot any grime or dust, and avoid having people over because you're afraid they'll judge you.

B. Keep it reasonably clean and clutter-free but, hey, you have better things to do than clean all the time.

C. Keep it spotless most of the time and stress out when it gets even slightly messy.

D. Vacuum twice a day, making sure that your vacuum leaves a pleasing pattern on the rug before you put it away. Anyone could eat off your floor, and your clothes in the closet are arranged by color and size, are on the same exact style of hanger, and all face the same direction at all times.

7. **You are learning a new skill and finding that you're not picking it up as quickly as you thought you would. You:**

A. Give up.

B. Try to identify ways to become more capable, and keep trying.

C. Get frustrated, put your head down, and work harder, inwardly berating yourself.

D. Hire a top coach to teach you this skill and rearrange your schedule so that you fix this problem now, once and for all, because, damn it, failure is not an option. Ever.

8. **What makes you feel self-conscious and embarrassed?**

A. You'd rather not answer this. You are uncomfortable just reading the question.

B. A few things, but nothing too serious or upsetting.

C. It's a long list because you're quick to beat up on yourself. Frankly, you're kind of insecure about how insecure you are and you think about your oversensitivities a lot.

D. "Wait, are you suggesting that there's something about myself that *doesn't* make me feel self-conscious and embarrassed?"

Scoring:

Mostly As: *Avoider.* You are afraid to step into your power and be criticized or make a mistake, so you avoid risks altogether, which is understandable. Your challenge is to aim for taking risks and owning your power to act rather than always delegating your power to others.

Mostly Bs. *Balanced.* You're responsible and accountable in a balanced way.

Mostly Cs: *Worrier.* You tend to worry too much and take too much responsibility for others, so watch your tendency toward perfectionism. Stop yourself from "fixing" situations and instead check in within and process your emotions.

Mostly Ds: *Perfectionist.* You are so anxious about not being in control that often you are out of control with your perfectionism! Your challenge is to work on trusting yourself and trusting in Spirit to support you. Regularly affirm *I love and accept myself just as I am. Spirit is nurturing me, supporting me, and looking out for me.*

We all walk between two pillars, one called I Create My Own Reality and one called I Have to Live Life on Life's Terms. The paradox of power is this: when we accept our powerlessness to control our lives, we reclaim our true power, which is the power of co-creating our reality with the help and influence of Spirit. When we reclaim this power, we remember our value, that we are each an irreplaceable child of Spirit.

Perfectionism makes us keep our eye on the clock and obsess over time, which exacerbates our anxiety, which drives us deeper into perfectionism and controlling behaviors. When you feel that time is closing in on you like the walls of a collapsing room, use the following exercise to create the perception that you have the time you need. Investing a few minutes in changing your perspective and easing your worries about time will actually save you time that you would've spent in unproductive agonizing.

SLOWING DOWN TIME

Take a long, deep breath, and focus on your breathing as you exhale, then inhale. Keep focusing on your breathing until you feel relaxed.

Now, imagine you see a large clock on the wall, the
old-fashioned kind with a second hand that runs around
the clock face. In front of it is a sort of elastic band of
energy about a foot long that shows you how much time you
have.

Just let the clock tick, tick, tick for a while. Breathe in
synchronously with its rhythm.

Slow your breathing, and imagine that the second hand begins
to slow down in synch with your breathing.

Look at the band of energy in front of the clock that was
supposed to be a measure of the time you have and watch it
expand as you relax and the second hand slows down.

How do you feel?

When you are ready, open your eyes.

DUMPING THE GARBAGE

As you've been writing in your Dumping Grounds journal, you've
surely generated a lot of trash—that is, thoughts and feelings that
don't serve your well-being but, instead, keep alive your negative
beliefs and painful emotions from the past. None of us is perfectly
self-compassionate, kind, loving, giving, and positive all the time.
Even Jesus lost his temper and kicked over a few tables, and called
some people "snakes." Sometimes, we just have to get all that anger,
sadness, and fear out of us and speak our truth, whatever it is at that
moment, however ugly it may be. I hope you've been using the Dumping Grounds journal to do this.

Now, however, it's important to let go of the harsh feelings and
judgments and focus on what you have learned and how you've grown.
At the end of the second step of this program, take out your journals
and have handy a yellow highlighting marker so you can highlight
some passages. As you read your journal entries, use your highlighter

to mark any passages that are "gems": insights that have value and can serve you in the future. Here and there, it's good to go back and reread these parts of your Dumping Grounds journal—and now you'll find them easily because they're in bright, sunny yellow. You'll want to write about your insights and the treasure you've found in your lessons in your Solutions and Insights journal. You'll be better able to track your real growth and progress, and less likely to sabotage yourself, when you've been able to keep these thoughts in separate physical spaces.

As you reread what you wrote, think about how much "weight" those thoughts and feelings had for you when you wrote them, and how much weight they have now. Does it seem like a lot of drama about something minor? Did you invest emotional energy in a situation or a thought or emotion that you now see really wasn't important?

Now, as you look at these passages, say aloud, *I release these thoughts and feelings with love and compassion for myself and everyone.* Imagine they are being taken to a garbage dump, then composted to serve as fertilizer for your Field of Dreams. In fact, nothing ever goes to waste! Take a moment to feel a sense of relief at having dumped the garbage.

As with Step One, you'll have some daily questions to answer in your Solutions and Insights journal, too. There aren't as many questions this week, so you'll only have to answer about two a day. If you finish up before the end of the week, that's okay. Just write in your journal about your feelings, how your day went, and what insights you're experiencing. Remember, you can vent as well, spilling all your hurt and anger onto the pages of your Dumping Grounds journal.

DAILY JOURNALING FOR STEP TWO:
OWN YOUR TRUTH

Write the answers to the following questions in your journal, and answer at least two questions a day.

1. Do you have an issue with trust? Anger? Jealousy? Envy? Procrastination?

2. Have you been dishonest with yourself or others in any way? Why?

3. Have you noticed that some of what you were feeling has little to do with you, that others in your environment have affected you?

4. Looking over what happened during Step One, what were you stimulated by?

5. Did you watch the news?

6. Was your work environment stressful?

7. Do the things that were bugging you for the past two weeks still affect you the same way today?

8. Would you choose to feel these things again?

9. If not, how would you choose to feel?

10. If you could change anything here, what would it be?

11. If you have no power to change anything here, can you imagine a higher power holding this burden for you? What if it was not a burden at all but only a perception of a burden?

12. What activities make you feel joyous and happy? What makes you laugh? How can you fit these activities into your life more often?

13. How do your usual surroundings (home, office) make you feel? How can you change your surroundings to make them more supportive of your joy?

14. In what ways does your body serve you well, despite any medical or health conditions you might have?

15. Write a letter of thanks to your body for how it has served you.

~~~~~~

Step Two is definitely challenging, but if you practice self-compassion and are kind to yourself, it will be easier. Be sure to "dump the garbage," sending it love and releasing it, at the end of the second week before you start on Step Three. Then your mind and heart will be clear and you'll be ready to enter the second half of the program.

Step Two, Week One: Exercises and Activities

- Be kind to yourself. (Remember KISS: kindness, IN-Vizion, salt, simplicity).
- IN-Vizion exercises as needed to help you manage your empathy overload and strong emotions.
- Morning journaling: What's your intention for today?
- 4:00 P.M. salt bath (or salt spritz, followed by a bath as soon as you can do it), during which you do use the EFT and affirmations, to speak your truth and process your feelings.
- Daily journaling: Answer about 2 exercises a day and journal about your resistance, feelings, insights, and experiences.
- Do each of the exercises within the chapter.
- Follow the simple plan of eating and movement. Continue to avoid physical stimulants and mental ones (such as the news and social media).
- Evening journaling: How did you do today? What is one thing you did right? What is one thing you're grateful for?

Step Two, Week Two: Maintenance Exercises and Activities

(By the way, you'll do these basic activities throughout this program and into the future).

- Be kind to yourself. (Remember KISS: kindness, IN-Vizion, salt, simplicity).
- IN-Vizion exercises as needed to help you manage your empathy overload and strong emotions.
- Morning journaling: What's your intention for today?
- Journal daily or every few days if you find journaling helps you to sort out your feelings.
- 4:00 P.M. salt bath (or salt spritz, followed by a bath as soon as you can do it), along with EFT to process your feelings.

- Follow the simple plan of eating and movement. Continue to avoid physical stimulants and mental ones (such as the news and social media).
- Evening journaling: How did you do today? What is one thing you did right? What is one thing you're grateful for?
- Dump the garbage at the end of week two. Do this by highlighting the "trash" with a pink marker and sending love and compassion to yourself as you reread what you've written. If you find "gems," or insights, highlight them in yellow so you can easily return to them.

KEEP IN MIND . . .

- During Step Two, you're likely to experience resistance as you start to realize you really do have a lot of work ahead of you, and that you can no longer deny that managing your porous boundaries has to be a priority if you're going to release the weight.
- Making the changes in this program will take you through the stages of denial, anger, bargaining, and sadness to acceptance. Recognize that transformation is a process and be patient with yourself at every stage.
- Establish a new habit of experiencing joy. Do what makes you happy and make feeling joyful a top priority. Redecorate and rearrange your space, getting rid of anything in it that doesn't support your joy.
- Establish a new habit of feeling gratitude toward your body. Listen to its needs and honor it with affirmations and by treating it well. Loving yourself means loving your body.
- Establish a new habit of connecting with Spirit. Use meditation, time spent in nature, prayer, and the Sacred Box. Then it will be

easier to feel the support of your higher power as you work the program.

- Perfectionism and stressing out about time are common detours because people who feel too much hate feeling out of control and are scared of criticism. Use the Slowing Down Time exercise to help you let go of these habits.

- When writing in your Dumping Grounds journal, feel free to vent about what is going on. You will release any "garbage" at the end of your processing week and highlight any insights that will build your confidence, esteem, and self-compassion whenever you reread them, and write about these in your Solutions and Insights journal.

Step Three: Reclaim Your Power to Choose ("There's a Difference Between a Compulsion and a Choice!")

You are halfway through the program. I'm guessing you no longer feel at the mercy of an out-of-control world, and you've stopped frantically swimming about in the turbulent seas of unrestrained emotions. At last, you can drop your hypervigilance and relax. It's much easier to make conscious decisions about what you're going to focus on and what actions you're going to take. Who wouldn't want to embrace the freedom to choose what to think about, feel, and do?

You will always have some strong emotions that seem to have a life of their own, which make it hard to think clearly and make good decisions, but by now you've realized you have more control over them than you thought you did. You let yourself feel anger or fear, but you don't exacerbate those emotions by allowing your thoughts to run wild—you stop and correct yourself. Those automatic, negative beliefs about yourself are being replaced by new, positive ones that you affirm daily. Inadequacy and low self-worth are on the wane. Enough of that!

You also have a better, more accurate perspective on your past battles with weight, food, and empathy overload. Now you see that you weren't armed with the wisdom you needed to disengage from fruitless obsessions over your weight, the shape of your body, or what you snacked on, so you aren't experiencing guilt or self-hatred as often as you used to. The old beliefs and feelings that go along with the guilt and self-hatred don't disappear overnight, but you have experienced their fading in intensity. Isn't it a relief to have quieter emotions?

When strong emotions do crop up, you now know what to do: you use the IN-Vizion Process to check in with yourself and see where you are, what's happening, and where you want to be. You know how to avoid empathy overload by doing your 4:00 P.M. salt baths, EFT, and affirmations, keeping the news and media stimulation to a minimum, and sticking to quiet foods rather than the noisy ones that trigger a strong, emotional reaction. Life is a lot calmer than it was just four weeks ago!

Now, in Step Three, you reclaim your power to consciously make good decisions instead of allowing your subconscious fear, anger, sadness, and agitation to take over your thoughts and whip up a frenzy of feelings that make you discombobulated. The first choice I know you'll want to make is to tame the whirlwind of emotion when it threatens to sweep you up. It's too stressful to be so reactive to what's going on around you and to get so agitated that you lose your power to make conscious choices.

One of the reasons people who feel too much become caught up in the emotional whirlwind is their habit of taking care of others. As I said earlier, because it's easy for you to tune in to others' emotions, you probably are a natural healer, nurturer, teacher, advocate, or caregiver (or a combination of these). Helping others is wonderful, but when you start to detour into enmeshment, codependency, and taking care of other people emotionally, it's a problem. You take on the weight of all their troubles and their painful emotions and hold them inside you while your rational mind tries to sort it out. Wouldn't it be better to turn all of this over to a higher power instead of turning it over in your head? You can also use the IN-Vizion Process to sort out your own emotions to deal with and let go of the rest, putting them in the Sacred Box.

KEEP HEALTHY BOUNDARIES:
DON'T SHARE THE GARBAGE!

Another choice you might want to make, now that you have greater clarity, objectivity, and self-compassion, is to use isolation in a positive way—not as a detour, but as a means of self-protection when you know you need a break from others' emotions. In other words, when you start to feel overwhelmed, you don't have to avoid everyone and take to your bed, but you also don't have to continue to subject yourself to other people's strong emotions. You can choose to temporarily isolate yourself from their emotions—or in some cases, from them.

Don't spend too much time around people who overstimulate you and distract you from your priorities, or around people who suck up your energy and attention because of their neediness or anger. These "energy vampires" don't necessarily mean to hurt you or wear you down. They may love you very much and want the best for you, but they are unable to understand that you truly can't handle all the emotion and upsetting information they dump on you.

One thing I hope you've learned by emptying, then sorting, your own garbage is that a lot of emotional crap swirls around inside of you until you get it out and away from you. You are probably drawn to other empathic people who have their own emotional agitation going on, in addition to empathy overload. Together, you and they are constantly exchanging energetic garbage. Understanding each other intellectually is great. But "understanding" each other by taking on each other's emotional turmoil is going to exhaust both of you. You need to clear out your own garbage before engaging with others, or you'll end up sharing it just as you would cold germs. If someone in your life is not ready to let you set some boundaries, and is hurt when you won't listen to the venting and dramas, you may have to avoid that person until she or he is ready to recognize that sharing anger, frustration, gossip, and the like are about as useful as sneezing in each other's faces.

Bond with people over solutions, not problems, and the gems of insight, not garbage. Instead of telling your sister-in-law about your hellish day at work, loading her up with every awful detail in order to trigger an empathetic reaction, just summarize what you experienced, without drama. Talk about what you learned, keep your sense of humor tuned up, and bond over how we all have "those days." The payoff of hearing "Oh, you poor thing!" is dwarfed by the payoff of not reliving every wretched moment of your day and then experiencing your friend's garbage dumping on you ("How awful! Let me tell you about how my terrible boss tortured me all day long—have I got a frustrating story to match yours!"). Stop the garbage flinging that has all of us, including you, covered in rotting banana peels and burnt toast scrapings.

Sometimes we have a sense that others have connected to us in an energetic way, almost as if we have a magnetic attraction to them (and their garbage!). We might want to unplug from the other's energy, but how do we do it? The Cord Unplugging exercise that follows offers a way to break the energy bonds that generate a feeling of being enmeshed with others.

CORD UNPLUGGING

Find a spot where you can be comfortable for about 5 to 10 minutes maximum.

Ask your body to relax. Feel each part of you release its tension—your neck, your shoulders, your arms, and so on. Next, ask your body to show you any place where you have connected to someone else's energy and created a feeling that the other person is inside your boundaries. Scan your body from your toes up to the top of your head. If you find a spot that seems to be enmeshed with energies outside of you, imagine that you have a little cord of energy hooked on to you in this place. Visualize it as a kind of electrical cord that, once unplugged from the outlet, can quickly retract back into the other person. See yourself unplugging the chord and having it recoil back into to whoever owns it.

Now, look to see if there's a cord coming from you that is plugged into someone else. If so, unplug it at their end and bring the cord back into yourself. Then seal yourself with a ball of light at each place where a cord was attached.

You will feel refreshed!

Now, did you notice any resistance to unplugging the cord?

Who were you plugged into? Who was plugged into you?

Why do you want to be bound to this person?

What, if anything, are you afraid to lose by unplugging?

What would it feel like to be separate and independent from him or her?

Ponder the answers to these questions, then take out your journal and write about your experiences doing this exercise.

～～～～～～～～～～～～～～～～～～～～～～～～～～～

WHOSE STUFF IS THIS?

One of my longtime clients, Elaina, was feeling overwhelmed and anxious, and she was giving me a detailed description about all that was going wrong in her life—a situation at her daughter's school, a fight with her husband, her stepson being arrested in another state. So, I had her do the IN-Vizion Process. I asked her where she was, and she described a finished basement in a large house where a toilet was overflowing. In her mind's eye, Elaina was alone in the basement, trying to unplug the toilet and find a way to clean up before anyone else came down and spotted the mess. She was grossed out by all the crap coming up from the toilet, and I told her to transport herself to the outside of the house. As soon as she found herself on the lawn, looking over at the house she had just escaped, she felt a sense of relief, and I told her to stay there for a few moments before reentering the basement. Then I asked her what was happening.

"I'm looking at the overflowing toilet and realizing, *This is not my shit! I don't have to clean it up!*" She felt herself walking up the stairs to the first floor of the house.

Not all of our landscapes are so obvious, but this is a perfect example of how we can become completely absorbed in trying to mop up shit and strategize the cleanup—without realizing it's not our shit. When Elaina used her rational mind to try to identify the shit, she intuitively understood that she was worrying too much about trying to get everyone in her child's school to become better educated on how to teach their children to manage their emotions so the bullying and teasing her daughter reported seeing would stop. (Remember, people who feel too much are often distressed when seeing others being bullied—that was the case with both Elaina and her highly sensitive daughter.) Elaina was able to see more clearly what her choices were and where her power lay—namely, in training her daughter to be bully-proof and to stand up for other children when they were being picked on, and in attending some school meetings about the bullying issue and expressing her opinion. What Elaina had to let go of was taking on responsibility for other people's denial, the other children's distress (which she kept imagining and worrying about), and fixing the problem single-handedly. She couldn't see where to draw boundaries when she was overwhelmed with empathy, and she actually could do more for the other children at the school by letting go of the useless obsessing over how they must feel being teased. An hour in the middle of the night spent losing sleep over their pain wasn't doing anything for anyone—the children or Elaina.

The IN-Vizion Process allows us to experience neutrality and nonreactivity. In this quiet state of observation, we can see more than our strong emotions will allow us to see. When we're upset, we're too focused on our feelings to notice that things aren't quite as bad as we make them out to be—and we've got others helping to address the problems that worry us. The story of "But I have to rescue those children or no one else will!" doesn't trap us because we see that helping to protect them from being hurt is a responsibility shared by many. We start to see evidence that we're not the only ones who care and are making an effort to help them. Perfectionistic, controlling, anxious behavior no longer has us in its grip.

However, the overflowing toilet in Elaina's IN-Vizion exercise represented more than the mess at Elaina's daughter's school. Elaina also told me that when she started fighting with her husband, he said, "I don't want to talk about this and sort out why you're mad at me and what I did. I think you're upset about something else." She was angry at his response, but sensed he was right, which is why she called me to sort it all out. I asked her about her stepson, and she said he had called four days before to tell her he had been arrested again for using drugs. Elaina had been avoiding calling her ex-husband and going to see her stepson, who was asking for her help.

I pointed out that the timing of all these problems was interesting: was it possible that she was overreacting to something in order to detour from her feelings about her stepson? In fact, that's exactly what was happening. It was less painful for Elaina to get herself all worked up about the hurt she imagined some children were feeling, and to avoid the pain of facing her drug-addicted stepson and alcoholic ex-husband again, as well as the pain of acknowledging that she could not control her stepson's addiction. She needed to feel like a successful rescuer, and the bullying incident at the school had been a distraction. Another distraction was her anger at her husband for pointing out that she was confused about her feelings.

Elaina needed to stop running away from *her* "stuff" and feel her emotions, and leave the rest for the Sacred Box. Once she made a conscious choice about how much to intervene with her stepson, and she spent some time crying about him, it was much easier for her to let go of her obsessive thoughts and her free-floating anger and anxiety about everything else.

In the past, Elaina would not have called me. She would have spent countless hours thinking about what was upsetting her and what to do, and would have lost sleep, eaten whatever was available instead of sticking with her commitment to eat healthfully, and completely lost herself in the detour of her emotional caregiving. With the storm quieted, she could exercise her power of choice. She chose to drop the argument with her husband, let her stepson walk his own path, and take specific actions to address the situation at her daughter's school without becoming an angel of righteousness swooping in with her sword of justice.

A VISION EMERGES FROM THE QUIET

From the quiet and calm of nonreactivity and neutrality, a vision of what your life could be can arise. Try the following exercise to help you envision the life you'd like to create for yourself.

CREATING AN EXPERIENCE BOARD

An Experience Board is like a dream board, in that you arrange photographs and words that evoke what you would like to bring into your life. But it's different in that the focus is on the *emotions* you want to create, not on the *things* you want to manifest (money, marriage, a thinner and healthier body, and so on).

Using a computer dream board program or an actual piece of poster board and photographs, create an Experience Board with images and words that express the emotions you would like to feel, such as joy, contentment, harmony, pride, confidence, and so on.

Every day, look at your Experience Board, and as your eyes focus on each image or word, feel the corresponding emotions rise in you. You can let your subconscious mind add to the image, too, making it into a mini movie. You might be surprised by the images your subconscious mind generates when you meditate on contentment or pride. If you find yourself resisting the emotion, or associating it with self-sacrifice instead of a balance between self-nurturing and caring for others, be glad that you made a discovery about your discomfort with that emotion. You may need to spend more time imagining how you might experience that emotion and what you could co-create in your life that would match up with that emotional experience. Can you imagine feeling confident even if you are doing something others might not understand or have an easy time accepting? Can you imagine feeling harmonious with someone without a drama of rescuer and rescued being played out between the two of you?

If you have trouble coming up with images, think about movies or television programs you have seen. Is there a sequence, scene, or image that evokes a powerful, positive emotion for you? Use it on your Experience Board and continue to work with the board, creating the emotions you would like to feel.

THE NEW YOU, EXERCISING THE POWER TO CHOOSE

Because we people who feel too much can quickly become overwhelmed by our emotions, we don't handle transition and uncertainty well. We like to know what we're dealing with, down to the last detail. It's what causes us to be perfectionists and to avoid change. We not only have our own anxiety to deal with, we also have the emotions of other people who are involved in the transition or change we are a part of—because those feelings seep in through our porous boundaries.

You might be eager to step into being a person who no longer detours through unhealthy caregiving of others, mindless eating, perfectionism, and so on. But are the people around you *ready* to support you? And can you handle their responses if they are jealous or angry toward you?

Let's say you are feeling excited about your new choice to nurture yourself by spending time alone, thereby enjoying activities that infuse you with optimism and energy, and this takes time away from your family. Your partner responds with resentment, your children become anxious because you aren't hovering over them catering to their every need, your mother is cynical and criticizes you for being selfish, and your best friend is encouraging (yay!). Of course, you want to take in your friend's encouragement and happiness for you, but how do you do that without taking on everyone else's emotions, which can intimidate and upset you?

Hmm, maybe you should spend more time with your best friend and avoid your family! Seriously, you do need to create boundaries with people who trigger your feelings of disempowerment and low self-worth. It's loving to listen to the feelings of the people you care about, but it's important to disengage from the negative emotional energy they generate in you. You can't always take on other people's anger or frustrations and you shouldn't have to.

If your partner is resentful of how much time you are now spending on self care, explain why your new habits are important to you. It may be that simply acknowledging that change in your life is difficult will be enough to get your partner on board. If the complaining or sighing continues, you're going to have to set a boundary: other people's feelings are theirs to manage and deal with, not to dump on you. The people who care about you ought to be happy for you if you are becoming healthier and more joyful. If they aren't, you need to talk to them about that and ask for their support.

If your family is having trouble adjusting to your new, less sacrificing self, they can use some of the techniques you've learned to manage their own difficult emotions as they transition to being less dependent on you. Talk through practical solutions if they're unhappy with how you aren't catering to them. Be creative about getting around any problems that come up. For example, maybe you and your partner can cook meals ahead of time so that when you come home on weeknights, you can take the 20 minutes for a bath without pushing back dinner for everyone.

Don't let yourself get drawn into the same unproductive, upsetting conversations again and again if your teenagers are working through their own uncertainty about the changes and are resistant to taking on more responsibility for themselves. Get your children involved in preparing healthier meals and make it a fun family time instead of a chore. Talk about what part of food preparation everyone likes best. One of my clients always loved to sit with her mother and snip the ends off of green beans when she was growing up; but later she learned that her own daughter would rather do just about anything than snip green beans, so was given the job of corn shucking and table setting. Trade off the food preparation chores and make sure everyone's preferences are heard.

At the end of a long day, anyone can be stressed out. When home, dinnertime should be nourishing to the body, mind, and spirit. If a family member or partner has to take a few minutes to process and let go of irritation, frustration, or deep funk, give the person leeway to do so, just as that person accommodates you by leaving you alone for 20 minutes while you do your salt bath and EFT. While chopping vegetables, setting the table, and cooking, talk about nonemotional topics. You might even play word games with the kids to keep the conversation light, so that you don't start taking on other people's emotions while you're around food. When you are eating, keep the conversation positive and encourage everyone to be mindful as they eat. Remark on how delicious the salad looks, or how tasty the in-season asparagus is. If anyone starts talking about how hard the day was, listen with sympathy but don't let him or her "dump garbage" all over your communal table! Make it a family rule that during meals, people can ask for emotional support but can't go into a rant about how awful today was.

Family time at the table should be about bonding, not about burdening each other. I remember family dinners, especially on Sundays, being highly valued in my home, but whenever there was tension between us or someone was in a bad mood, it was hard to eat. Still, it made us all closer to break bread together. If I could go back in time, I would teach everyone how to process his or her emotions without bringing them to the table and serving them up with the soup.

The old habit of "balancing" your needs with your family's by flushing yours down the drain and endlessly catering to others has come to an end. You have the choice not to slip back into that behavior. Set rules for sharing meal preparation and eating together without bringing in drama.

As for what you eat, you might hear a lot of noise when you stop cooking, buying, and serving foods that aren't healthy for you. One of my weight-loss clients told her husband to keep his cookies and chips in his garage workshop, out of her sight. He needed to lose weight as well, but it wasn't her responsibility to get him to cut out the junk food. They stopped having regular conflicts about food once she set the boundary and the noisy foods weren't around to tempt her.

As you're make changes in how you eat, you are also making changes in how much you are isolating yourself. Welcome back to civilization! However, don't be surprised if a few people don't greet your return with welcoming arms. They may not trust that you really do care about connecting with them emotionally, and that you're not going to avoid intimacy and isolate again. It may take some time to rebuild your relationships with your partner, your siblings, your kids, and so on. Again, be sure to do your daily journal writing and the exercises in this chapter to begin imagining what your relationships will look like; now, you aren't disappearing on people as soon as they become emotional, or engaging in codependent behavior that has them feeling smothered and controlled.

In a sense, you're reentering that middle school, awkward age again when you try on new behaviors and discover who you are, reclaiming pieces of yourself that got lost along the way or that you were afraid to look at. Remember discovering your rebellious self for the first time? Did you hold on to that aspect of yourself, or did you run from it, afraid of what might happen if you allowed yourself to step off the straight-and-narrow path? Now that you are older, wiser, stronger, and armed with many techniques for managing your painful emotions, you can take another look at the aspects of yourself that you were afraid to claim or hold on to. You can choose to reincorporate them into your life. Rebelliousness can take many forms in your life, some of which can be very positive. How might it manifest in your life now, if you choose to reclaim it?

ASSERTING YOURSELF: YOU DON'T HAVE TO BE ALLERGIC TO CONFRONTATION!

To some of you, assertive behavior may come naturally, but to many of you, the people-pleasing habit is so engrained that you would rather die of salmonella poisoning than tell the waitress to return your undercooked eggs to the kitchen—you don't want to hurt anyone's feelings. Does reading the word *confrontation* make your stomach tighten? I know it does for me. I hate confrontation and will do anything to avoid it, but that approach has got me into a lot of trouble in the past. It took me many years to heal from being gang-raped at age 19, which set in motion a strange possum-playing behavior when faced with someone else's anger or drama. It took me years to stand up for myself when I was being abused because I had been so traumatized by the event; it was easier to just shut down and ignore whatever was happening.

I could write a whole other book about all of that, but suffice it to say that people pleasing can be a survival skill that the subconscious mind has mastered. It takes a lot of practice and self-compassion to retrain your brain to allow your subconscious mind to speak its piece—*Ooo, are you sure you want to do that? Remember what happened in the past!*—and have your conscious mind override it: *Yes, but that's not going to dictate what I do in the present or future. Thanks for the warning, but I'm safe right now, and making a good decision.* Whether you grew up experiencing abuse or trauma, or you simply are oversensitive, you probably hate confrontation just as much as I do. Unfortunately, avoiding confrontation often creates the very situations you are trying to avoid.

My client Douglas was a lifelong people pleaser. He would do anything to avoid making someone angry, resentful, jealous, hurt, or sad. He didn't understand that we are *not* responsible for other people's feelings, just for our own behavior. Douglas would not tell his business partner bad news, even when it was important that he be aware of problems. He hid the fact that one of their company's clients was asking for far more than Douglas and his partner had agreed to in their contract with the client. In fact, the client threatened to pull his business if they didn't provide the extra services. Douglas worked long hours to keep the client happy and he hid from his partner how bad the situation was. Finally, he was so overworked and stressed out that he made a major blunder and the client refused to pay his bill anyway.

Douglas's partner was stunned to find out what was going on, and he nearly ended his partnership with Douglas over the deception. They had many options early on: they could have let go of the customer, could have tried reasoning with him and found a compromise, spoken to their lawyer about the contract. But Douglas removed all those options by avoiding a confrontation with either the client or his partner. In the end, they were both furious with him!

Our fear of confrontation is a major factor in our high tolerance for insanity. Many of us put up with far more craziness than the average person would, either because "crazy" feels normal to us, given our backgrounds, or because we are sensitive to other people's pain, shame, and embarrassment. How can we possibly confront the person or reject him? What if he gets mad at us? The thought is stomach churning. We're equally unnerved if we're confronted by the person because we didn't call or follow through on the foolish promise we made earlier, when we were willing to do anything to avoid confrontation or disapproval.

As you stop taking on the weight of other people's emotions, it becomes easier to confront people nicely and right away, instead of waiting until a situation is disastrous. It becomes easier to take risks and ask for what you need *and* what you want. You can simply *want* more information, more control, and more predictability, and you can ask for it without going into a long explanation of why you need and deserve it. Assertiveness means not launching into a dissertation whenever you make a request. For instance, don't tell the waitress about your fear of salmonella and your low immunity because you just got over the flu (even though it's a white lie you've invented to make a stronger case for the righteousness of your cause). Don't apologize profusely for the inconvenience. Just say, "Excuse me. These eggs are undercooked and I'd like to send them back. Thanks." That's it—no speech or bowing and scraping required. Afterward, if you find yourself overstimulated and hyper because you finally stood up for yourself, or you are stressing out because even though the waitress was nice, maybe the cook hates you now, *stop*. Use your techniques for letting go of the empathy and emotional overload.

Let's consider the worst case: the other person responds badly to your assertiveness. Don't give her feelings more weight than she does, then take those feelings on! You might ignore the mild resistance or ask for more information. I think many sensitive people have gotten into the habit of being intimidated by any grumbling or eyeball rolling from the person who is resisting. Ignoring mild resistance can often be a good choice, regardless of what your gender is or who is unhappy with your request, especially if you know that person well and you know what you are asking is reasonable. Remember, *nonreactivity* and *neutrality* are your goals when confronted with someone's anger, frustration, or fear—or grumbling.

Maybe you decide to ask why this person seems to resent your request. Notice how I said *seems* to resent it. You might be misreading her hesitation or her frown. You may be intuitive, but you're not necessarily right all the time about others' subtle feelings! Be open to the possibility that you're wrong.

If you're not misreading, then breathe deeply and slowly while the other person is talking. You can handle this temporary discomfort and use your cleaning techniques afterward to shed any emotional weight of hers that you take on.

Let's say the person isn't interested in finding common ground and in resolving the conflict, but just starts to dump his garbage on you. Saying "I'm sorry you feel that way" acknowledges and honors his feelings without taking responsibility for them. "I'm sorry" doesn't mean, "I'm sorry, it's all my fault, you should be angry with me! How horrible I am! Oh, I feel like dirt!" It just means, "I feel compassion for you because you are upset and I'd like to express that to you."

Once you've expressed "I'm sorry you feel that way," then you can make your decision. Are you going to remain in place, being dumped on? Are you going to politely excuse yourself or change the subject? It's okay to cut him off. He can come back to you and talk to you again at some point when he's dumped his garbage and ready to be sensitive to your feelings. The choice of what to do when someone is being cruel to you is yours now. You're no longer going to be automatically sucked into the vortex of other people's strong emotions. There is a breath, a moment, in which you access your neutrality, observe what's happening, and make a nonreactive choice about going to the landscape that person is creating. Maybe the stormy fields where he is raging is *his* landscape to visit and learn from, not yours. You do not have to be in his emotional space.

What if you confront someone and the other person denies there is anything wrong and pouts? Again, you can try to get more information— maybe she is afraid to tell you why she is upset—or you can ignore it. It's up to you to decide what to do. You're not responsible for passive-aggressive behavior. For instance, the response, "Oh, I'm not upset. Why would I be upset?" delivered with teeth clenched and a glare is passive-aggressive. If you want to be assertive, you might say, "Then why are your teeth clenched and why are you looking at me like that?"

Sometimes, it feels good to shine a big light on the social lie. Other times, it feels good to let it go and let that person figure out how she wants to handle her emotional response. You are not a garbage dump anymore, and you don't get paid to be everyone's personal psychologist and social worker. Let her work through her tangle of emotions on her own. Then you can step back and cleanse your emotional field.

Do you get the picture? Do you want to step into it? It's possible, but be patient with yourself during this awkward stage. Just as there is no quick-fix diet, there's no quick fix to your habit of bending over backward for people and forgetting where you end and they begin. You are creating a new relationship with yourself and with food at the same time you are creating new relationships with people. Evolution is messy and happens unevenly. Some days, you will have breakthroughs that astound you, and other days you will think, "I'm never going to get this!" You will. Change happens, just not as smoothly and as quickly as you would like it to.

In the meantime, keep planning the new life you are creating for yourself. What would you like to bring into it? Here's another exercise to help you get some ideas.

SHOPPING LIST FOR YOUR NEW LIFE

Start a shopping list for your new life, as if you could simply pop over to the store and pick up what you would like, with someone else covering the bill. If you weren't thinking about all the obstacles between you and the life you'd like for yourself, what would you "pick up"?

Would you want to bring in more time with friends? What would you do with them? Would you talk over lunch or drinks, or while walking your dogs to the dog run together?

What opportunities would you slip into your cart, for use when you are ready? Would you want an opportunity to exercise socially without feeling that everyone is staring at you or judging you? What would that opportunity look like?

What kind of food would you pick up? What cooking skills would you simply purchase and start using?

What clothes will you wear? What will they say about you?

What job or jobs will you have? What responsibilities will you take on? Will the work you do be fulfilling? Will the people you work with be flexible and respectful of your needs? What will that look like? Will you collaborate with them or compete with them?

As you draw up your list, if you feel hesitation about acknowledging what you want for yourself, stop. Get in touch with why you feel that situation is off-limits to you. Use the IN-Vizion process to learn more about why you don't believe you can have what you desire.

~~~~~~

DON'T FILL UP THE CART WITH DRAMA

Have you ever been to one of those big warehouse clubs or bargain stores and found yourself dumping into the cart anything that catches your eye because, hey, it's a bargain? Then you get to the cash register, hear the total, and fall over in shock.

We do this metaphorically when we let go of what we no longer want to hold on to, but we don't do the work of planning what to bring in instead. When the kids leave for college, or an aging and needy parent dies, it would make sense to regroup and start thinking about the next chapter of life; but too often, people who feel too much can't bear the uncertainty of not knowing what comes next. Rather than enjoying the process of planning for something new, and trying out new activities, and simply resting, we tend to rush out and find drama and stimulation to fill the void. Whatever caregiving opportunity catches our eye, we grab it and throw it in the cart. In this way, we detour away from our grief over the end of an important part of our lives, and the feelings we pushed aside for months or years while tending to the business at hand. There's a certain comfort in knowing that we can handle whatever comes our way, multitasking and staying completely focused on the latest crisis. Quiet and stillness make us want to scream.

In the void, difficult feelings come up. Maybe this happens because we sense we are finally safe enough to face the anger, sadness, or fear that we've stuffed into the back closet of our minds in order to avoid the discomfort. A few years back, I had a client who had lost her husband of thirty years, and she was shocked at how much anger was coming up for her from who knows where. What was she so furious about? She said her husband was loving, supportive, a good provider—and yet, all those years he was alive, she never confronted him about her needs, and conformed to all his wishes and quirks. The amount of anger that was bubbling up to the surface scared her. Who knew that garbage was rotting away inside her? Much as she was tempted to distract herself with some dramas involving her adult children, what she most needed to do is accept that she was in transition and needed to work through her anger. She had to dump the garbage, sort through it for any gems of insight, and begin planning the next stage of her life.

We live in such a fast-paced world that most of us have become used to running nonstop, from the moment we wake up to the moment we fall asleep at night. Transition, uncertainty, and contemplation all make us itch. At these times, it's helpful to work with a coach or therapist to help avoid the detour of stimulation and stay focused on resolving the past and imagining what we'd like to experience in the future. We can't let the uneasy feelings we have during transitions make us reactive to noisy foods and situations that aren't ours to take on.

KEEPING IT LIGHT

You know it feels good to laugh, but did you also know it's good for your health? Laughing is stimulating, but it also relaxes you and relieves tension and stress. It opens your blood vessels, increasing circulation and possibly preventing heart attacks. Laughter seems to boost your immune system and even ease physical pain. So embrace your inner clown. Choose to laugh, to lighten up and to see the humor in situations.

People who feel too much often have a habit of letting their perfectionism and fear of being seen as inadequate or foolish keep them tightly wound and afraid of laughing and joking around. Start imagining ways you might bring laughter into your life. What would it look like to be "silly" or "goofy" and not take in anyone's disapproval or negative judgment?

Humor is honest—the court jester was the one fellow who could tell the king what was really going on, and he was funny because he was willing to say what no one else would. When you laugh at your weaknesses and failings, though, it's empowering. You tell the truth and it doesn't devastate you after all.

It's wonderful to be able to laugh at yourself, and it may take you some time to develop the confidence to do so. Find the part of you that can let out a big belly laugh and guffaw until your eyes water and you gasp for breath. You can start by watching a funny movie, television show, or video, or reading something that makes you laugh out loud. Pay attention to how good it feels to cut loose and laugh, and how much lighter you feel afterward; then journal about it. What emotions come up after you laugh? Do you feel guilty or ashamed? What thoughts come up for you? Are there thoughts or beliefs that would better serve you? Think about turning those new thoughts into affirmations and add them to the affirmations you use during your 4:00 P.M. salt baths.

Bring more laughter into your life. And the next time you feel anxious and upset, roar "Grrrr!" and pretend to tear your hair out or cross your eyes and make a face. It's hard to hold on to anger and fear when you are being ridiculous.

THE DETOUR OF CARETAKING

As I said earlier in the book, because you're so tuned in to others' emotions, you have a natural talent as a healer, caretaker, or nurturer and can help others who are distressed; besides, you feel driven to help them. We people who feel too much can't stand to see other people in pain. It makes us deeply uncomfortable, so we feel we have to assist them and help them in their situations—right now before we go crazy. That desire to help someone else is really a way to protect ourselves from pain, too. We can get into big trouble owing to this urge to save the world from suffering; we take care of people in order to ground ourselves, and we can overstep their boundaries, become codependent, and burn ourselves out in the caretaking.

When the desire to help crosses into codependency, when you're actually taking responsibility for other people's emotions and protecting the person from the consequences of her choices, you may unconsciously have too much of a stake in being needed. You might be holding on tenaciously to an identity of the dutiful child, the good girl, the one who can always be counted on, the one whose is endlessly giving, and so on. I have a client who prides herself in being there for everyone all the time, regularly complains about how she has no time for herself, but balks when it's suggested that not setting healthier boundaries with others may be contributing to her being overweight. Surely the metaphoric weight of the world that she has taken on might very well be showing up on her hips?

For people who feel too much detouring into über-caretaking mode, the question is why we do it. My client was agitated and fearful with the thought of not taking care of others. She wondered aloud, *Who will I be if I'm not the one to solve everything for everyone? Why would people want me around? What would my place be?* Her radically honest questions about what it would mean to change were particularly painful for her to ask since no one wants to admit he or she might not have intrinsic value, that it's enough just to be who we are, without endlessly giving and giving. And it's so much easier to consider someone else's plight, worrying and talking about the person, than being in your own skin. Perhaps our greatest asset as people who feel too much is that we pride ourselves in caring for others; but when we detour into caretaking, our sensitivity, empathy, and intuition can cause us heartache.

I can't stress enough the power of the subconscious mind in determining our feelings and behaviors. The subconscious influences your choices far more than you think. It may be pushy and even obnoxious, dominating you so often, but at least the subconscious also knows what's going on! What do you do in a pinch to remind yourself that you have the power of choice, you are not engulfed by agitation, and you are in control? Is it really possible to be neutral and nonreactive, to not become overwhelmed by or obsessed with your emotional response to something that's happening? Yes!

The IN-Vizion Process allows you to disengage from your emotions by turning them into a landscape that you can observe and, maybe more important, *exit* at any time. It may be uncomfortable in those stormy fields, but if you know you have the power to survey them and make your escape whenever you choose, your fear and anger won't engulf you. Remember, when you're in a primitive panic response, and you feel as if there's a rhinoceros charging at you, you've got very little blood flow to the front of your brain where you can tolerate your difficult feelings and quiet them enough to plan your next move and make a good decision. You have to calm your fight-or-flight response, and the IN-Vizion Process can help with that. Then, you won't feel the need to detour to disordered eating and ground yourself with food, or manage your emotions by becoming overly involved in someone else's life.

The IN-Vizion Process will help you shift out of reactivity at any time, but if you keep practicing with it, you'll start to see that you're not as quick to pick up the gauntlet thrown down by someone else. Instead, you may feel rising irritation or frustration, but you'll know that you have a choice not to become immersed in those emotions—or anyone else's emotions. I think we often don't realize how much practice it takes to establish new habits, and then we get down on ourselves and give up. You're not going to be the Zen Buddha when someone hurts your feelings or treats you badly, but you're not going to spin out of control instantly, either. It will take practice to automatically remember in those moments of extreme agitation that you can shift gears and awaken your observing self and your power of choice.

If you want to share in someone's fear or anger, empathizing with that person so that he feels heard, you will still have that choice—but you can make that choice consciously. The question is how attached you are to the drama. Can you imagine what your relationships would be like if you *sympathized* with others, expressing compassion toward them instead of taking on the weight of their emotions? Most of us don't take the time to think about what our lives might be like if we followed through and enacted the changes we say we'd like to make. Take a little time to do the next exercise and explore how different your life could be.

WHAT MY LIFE WOULD BE

Imagine that you were to change your whole life, not just your body. What would be the quality of your relationships? If you were to stop becoming enmeshed with people, immersing yourself in their dramas, what would your life be like? Take some time to answer these and the following questions. You might want to do more than one session, writing in your journal for up to a half hour at a time.

- If you could clear away and unplug from any and all unwanted or burdensome energy, what would that feel like?

Go back and review your nighttime notes. Make a list summarizing everything you have done well since you began this program. Pay special attention to anything you've done that has served your higher good. Read the list. Write about how you feel.

- How do you feel about continuing the program?
- What are you afraid of?
- What would it look like if you didn't hold on to that fear?
- Can you love yourself enough, and trust in a higher power to love you when you can't?
- Imagine yourself sitting in the hand of your higher power, surrounded by unconditional love. Now how do you feel?

Once you've reclaimed your power, that old feeling of "Where do I end and you begin?" fades. You have a stronger sense of yourself as an individual with choices, so you can stop yourself when you feel you're becoming engulfed in a wave of someone else's emotions. Reconnecting with others is a less frightening prospect. What's more, now that you know practical ways to deal with your painful emotions, it becomes easier to reconnect with your body, thoughts, and feelings. You don't have to isolate or insulate yourself with excess weight that keeps people away. You can start to look into the mirror and see your whole body, instead of keeping your gaze at neck level or above, and you can reconnect with your spirituality in a way that feels right to you. Other people's disapproval or anger doesn't have to permeate your energy field. It's going to get easier and easier to avoid the noisy foods that falsely promise, "Eat me and you'll feel better!" I hope you're already feeling freer and lighter as we go into Step Four: Reconnect Without Losing Yourself.

DAILY JOURNALING FOR STEP THREE: RECLAIM YOUR POWER TO CHOOSE

Write the answers to the following questions in your journal. Allow at least 20 minutes for this process each day for 7 days, and answer about two questions a day.

1. What would your life look like if you released the weight of the world?

2. What would your life look like if you didn't rush in to save other people from the consequences of their actions? What would it look like to let others make mistakes without you trying to intervene?

3. Who might you be if you weren't taking responsibility for other people's emotions? What would you do with all that time you would free up, time you currently spend worrying about others?

4. What would you like to do that you never seem to have time for? What would it look like if you did have time for it?

5. What would your relationships look like if you set healthy boundaries and said no to people who want to dump their garbage on you? What would their initial response be? What would happen if you stood your ground?

6. Do you think you have to take on responsibility for other people and their feelings in order to be a good and lovable person? If so, why?

7. What would your life look like if you were a good and lovable person with healthy boundaries in your relationships?

8. What are you afraid of?

9. What do you want to create for yourself?

10. What emotions would you like to experience regularly?

11. What would your life look like if you gave up your anger and resentment? Would you still be a good, caring person?

12. What would your life look like if you forgave yourself for your failures, and the people you care about for hurting you?

13. What would happen if you found space on your to-do list for self-nurturing? What would your days look like?

14. What are you holding on to? What would it feel like to let it go? What would it feel like once it was gone from your life?

15. How does your oversensitivity manifest in your life? How would you like it to manifest in your life? In other words, if oversensitivity and an ability to be deeply empathetic were a gift and never a burden, what would your life look like?

Step Three, Week One: Exercises and Activities

- Be kind to yourself. (Remember KISS: kindness, IN-Vizion, salt, simplicity).

- IN-Vizion exercises as needed to help you manage your empathy overload and strong emotions.
- Morning journaling: What's your intention for today?
- 4:00 P.M. salt bath (or salt spritz, followed by a bath as soon as you can do it), during which you do use the EFT and affirmations to speak your truth and process your feelings.
- Daily journaling: Answer about two questions a day and journal about your resistance, feelings, insights, and experiences.
- Do each of the exercises within the chapter.
- Follow the simple plan of eating and movement. Continue to avoid physical stimulants and mental ones (such as the news and social media).
- Evening journaling: How did you do today? What is one thing you did right? What is one thing you're grateful for?

Step Three, Week Two:
Maintenance Exercises and Activities

- Be kind to yourself. (Remember KISS: kindness, IN-Vizion, salt, simplicity).
- IN-Vizion exercises as needed to help you manage your empathy overload and strong emotions.
- Morning journaling: What's your intention for today?
- Journal daily or every few days if you find journaling helps you to sort out your feelings.
- Dump the garbage at the end of the second week of Step Three.
- 4:00 P.M. salt bath (or salt spritz, followed by a bath as soon as you can do it), along with EFT to process your feelings.
- Follow the simple plan of eating and movement. Continue to avoid physical stimulants and mental ones (such as the news and social media).

- Evening journaling: How did you do today? What is one thing you did right?
- End of week: Dump the garbage.

KEEP IN MIND . . .

- When overwhelmed by emotions, don't focus on everyone and anything. Get in touch with what's really bothering you and put the problems that aren't a priority into the Sacred Box, trusting that Spirit will take care of them while you address your own emotional storm.
- Don't "bond over bitching." Don't share garbage with others by venting. Share solutions and emotional support.
- Create an Experience Board to begin imagining the emotional experiences you'd like to have.
- Exercise your power of choice. Be compassionate toward those who are uncomfortable with your new choices, but don't give your power of choice to them. Let them learn to adjust to your new way of operating.
- Assert yourself, without apologies or justifications and explanations. Practice letting go of the need to imagine, *What is that person going to think of me?* and taking on his or her emotions.
- Start to think about what you want to bring into your life to replace your old patterns of enmeshing with others and detouring away from your discomfort. Actually picture yourself filling a shopping cart with the emotional experiences you'd prefer to have.
- Don't fill your cart with drama. Remember, you have the choice about what you want to bring into your life. You don't *have* to choose to bring in drama that stimulates you and churns up

your emotions, distracts you, and drives you to detour away from healthy eating.

- Keep it light. Learn to laugh at the everyday things that would otherwise frustrate you.
- Continue to use the IN-Vizion Process and explore your inner emotional landscape as an observer who can make choices. The more you do this, the easier it will be to avoid reactivity and avoid detouring into caregiving for others, practically or emotionally.

Step Four: Reconnect Without Losing Yourself ("I Don't Have to Leave the Party After All!")

Are you successfully managing your porous boundaries much of the time? If you start to feel overwhelmed by a tangle of emotions twisting and turning inside of you, and you are tempted to ground yourself with food, now you know what to do besides open the pantry or refrigerator.

It's easier now for you to look honestly at the choices you have been making; your self-compassion muscle has been toned and you know that your weight issues aren't just about food. When you began this program, you probably would have instantly launched into a tirade against yourself if you had overeaten, but you don't do that anymore—or if you do, you cut yourself off very quickly. Remember, it's possible that once in a while you'll have a moment when you fall back into the old, reactive behavior; but now that your self-worth is greater and your habits are different, you have reclaimed the power of choice.

I shared with you my moments of struggle that I still have, but one thing is certain: loving yourself, accepting yourself, having self-esteem, feeling safe inside your own skin is worth more than a number on the scale. And, the longer you practice this program, the easier it will be to drop the excess weight and be in the world without being consumed and overwhelmed by it.

Take a moment and think about how much progress you have made. If you feel you've gotten stuck, and can't move forward because you're resisting the program, don't quit! Keep using the techniques you've learned, and you will prime yourself to recognize what's holding you back and what you need to do for yourself.

As you begin this final step of the program, you have come to claim your power to create neutrality and nonreactivity. Part of your consciousness is able to separate out from what you are craving and feeling, which allows your rational mind to think about what choices you want to make. Mindless, disordered eating is no longer the norm. Now it's time to reconnect—to your body, your feelings, your beliefs, and even to other people. Neutrality and nonreactivity make it much easier to let go of the old detouring behaviors of isolation and enmeshment and to build healthy relationships and boundaries. You don't have to be afraid of feeling overwhelmed and powerless anymore. Whatever you find or experience when reconnecting, you can handle it now. What a relief that is!

Often, we people who feel too much isolate ourselves, not just by avoiding other people but also by disconnecting our mind from our emotions, or ignoring our body's needs. We become easily overwhelmed by how we feel, and by our thoughts, so we cut off the part that's hurting—the body that needs movement and good food, the emotions that need expressing, the thoughts that might cause us discomfort. Mind, body, and spirit can come together now as you unite all the pieces of yourself—no more being the highly successful, ever efficient businessperson who secretly binges and purges, or the compassionate counselor who flies into rages and then feels guilty. You are going to own all the parts of yourself, even the ones you'd like to deny, and you will incorporate them into the beautiful, complex person that is you.

Let's look at the pieces of yourself that you have compartmentalized so that you could ignore them when your feelings were too intense, and see how you can integrate them into who you are now.

RECONNECTING TO YOUR BODY

When I was younger, I had completely unrealistic and limited ideas about what my body should look like. I hated that I couldn't get my body to conform to the shape I wanted it to be. Even when I was at my slimmest, my frame still had a stocky quality—big boobs, short waist, long yet thick legs. We used to joke that I got the hearty Polish and Yugoslavian genes and my lean teeny sister got the aristocratic French genes. Until the age of 14, I was a tomboy, athletic, and not particularly pretty, until I blossomed at 15. I never saw myself reflected in any magazine photos while growing up. All the women who were presented as beauty to aspire to were models obviously out of reach for me. Brigitte Bardot, Sophia Loren, and Marilyn Monroe were my favorites, but then they quickly faded into the distance and I had Twiggy and Veruschka to look at in magazines in the '60s, then gorgeous, thin, long-haired hippy girls in the '70s. I felt I had to look like the perky Charlie's Angels, especially Farrah Fawcett, who was blond and slender, while I could boast of neither attribute. So growing up, I never could see how I could fit in—at least, in the beauty department. I wish the Kardashian girls had been born thirty years earlier, as it would have made my life a lot easier if they were my TV or magazine models. Love 'em or hate 'em, their curvy bodaciousness sure makes me happy, given that I have a similar look.

Nowadays, software makes it so easy to retouch photographs and video, to such an extreme that even fashion models don't look like their pictures do. It's becoming harder and harder to remember the difference between what a real body and face look like compared to the highly altered images we see around us constantly. I feel for the young women—and men—who grow up thinking that their bodies are supposed to resemble these highly altered images. And it's not just the fashion models who are ultra-thin—now, actresses, actors, and models in health magazines also present body images that few people can attain.

LOVE YOUR AGING BODY

Several years ago, I was at my most toned and trimmed because I was managing my emotions, eating well, and working out with a personal trainer five days a week. Well, I was 42 years old back then, and now I am twelve years older and things have changed—my lifestyle, menopause, and so much more. As I'm aging, I'm learning to love my changing body just as it is each day, and I've made a conscious decision not to go back to such intense physical exercise. I train just three times a week and do light cardio the rest of the time. At this point in my life—most of the time—I am happy with how I look because I'm happy overall.

Have I thrown out those skintight jeans I wore ten years ago? Okay, I am not perfect. If I'm really going to let it all hang out for you all, I will admit that I keep a secret stash in my closet of my favorite skinny clothes, which says more about my squirreling habits than anything else! But I will say, wholeheartedly, that I am free of the obsession over my body and my weight. Other than the occasional episode, which only comes on when I don't practice what I preach, I am light-years away from that 219-pound young woman shrieking in the bathroom because she didn't recognize the image of the naked fat girl in the mirror coming out of the shower!

My good spirits show in my face and in how I carry myself. Twelve years ago, it took an enormous amount of effort to maintain that weight and muscle tone, and I don't want to spend all my time sculpting my body anymore. Health and stamina are very important to me, but I have a lot to do, and heavy exercise is too intense for my aging body and its joints. I don't want to get injured or exhaust myself pushing my body the way I used to. Whenever I do feel that sense of dread in trying on clothes or being around some of my naturally thin-bodied friends, it lasts seconds, if it happens at all. I remind myself how far I've come and how who I am really has nothing to do with what my body looks like in comparison to others.

I have a menopausal tummy, which is actually pretty flat—just wider. I work out and eat cleanly, and I accept and love my belly as it is today because it's a part of who I am and it serves me well. One of my class participants wrote a letter to her belly telling it how fabulous it is. In fact, if you're menopausal, you may not realize that your belly is helping you. As Julia Ross says in her book *The Diet Cure*, "Muscle burns fat for a living; it uses fat as fuel for its activity. But we put on menopausal fat for an excellent reason: we need it so that we can feed our adrenals the special fat-storage estrogen, called estrone, that helps them replace the estrogen that used to come from our ovaries." So every morning, I stroke my favorite orange-scented cream from The Body Shop all over my menopausal belly and tell "her" how beautiful she is, thanking her for doing her job.

NO MORE OBSESSING OVER IMPERFECTIONS

If you are still struggling with body image, don't underestimate how much you're being affected by doctored media images and unrealistic expectations about looking like a still-growing adolescent when you're well past that age. Avoid false media images as much as possible, and try to spend some time around people your age who are not covering up their bodies—at the beach, at a dance class, a pool, or health club. If you go to these places, you are probably used to looking at the toned, ultra-thin bodies and ignoring how many bodies look like yours. It's important to remember how easily our perceptions can become distorted; check yourself when you start obsessing about how your body isn't perfect. Ah, there goes that perfectionism again!

The Weight Loss for People Who Feel Too Much program is designed to free you from your obsessions about your body and weight. Liberation comes from radical self-acceptance. When you let go of the weight of self-judgment or self-hatred, you make it easier for your body to also let go of the physical weight you are carrying. And your body will know where it wants to be! Your body is wise and you must trust it! I couldn't lose an ounce until I began loving myself and my body when I was at my heaviest. While I was afraid of it and hated it the worse it got, the more the weight stuck to me like glue. Dieting never worked.

Self-acceptance, self-love, setting healthy boundaries, and eating for health were what did it.

How do you feel about your body? Can you imagine loving it as it is right now? Are you starting to give up the battle to bully it into being something it can't be, into a shape and size you can't obtain, because of your age and your genetics? If not, take a look at some photographs of your relatives, particularly pictures from the past, or even photographs of people of your age who are in your ethnic group. Your genes have a strong influence on whether you are short and stocky, tall and big boned, or petite and round. When you look at people who share DNA with you, you realize why that youthful dream of a bubble butt or perfect abs was always unrealistic, given your body type. That doesn't mean you can't love your body exactly as it is right now.

Even if you have health problems that frustrate you because they cause you pain or fatigue, or limit you in some way, you have to learn to love your body as it is in any moment. Self-compassion means embracing your physique now, not as it once was, not as you hope it will be someday.

When you catch yourself saying cruel things to yourself about your shape, your face, or your body, stop, take a breath, and say some affirmations about how strong, wonderful, loving, and beautiful your body is. The following exercise will drive the point home because you do it while you are caressing your body.

I LOVE MY BODY!

After a salt bath, dry off, and while your body is still warm and moist, take some moisturizer and begin to rub it into your body, slowly. Imagine yourself as a sensual goddess, poised next to a beautiful fountain or lagoon, the warm breeze gently rippling over you as you sit nude, the picture of perfection. Say to yourself:

I am a work of art, a beautiful physical creation. I love myself. I love my body.

I love my skin, my beautiful skin that keeps me healthy,

protecting me. I love my hands, and all they do to serve me. They allow me to reach for what I want. I love my feet, which hold me up.

Continue naming the parts of you as you rub the moisturizer into them, naming what they do for you. End with:

My body is healthy and strong. My blood moves easily and effortlessly through my body. I draw in breath, deeply, nourishing my body, giving life to every cell.

My heart beats, keeping me alive and in this beautiful, wonderful, healthy body.

My body is a gift. My body is a divine expression of life.

I am beautiful.

~~~~~~

One thing I've noticed is that we obsess about our weight and bodies because we are detouring away from some other difficult emotion. If you feel taken advantage of at work, or your romantic partner isn't treating you right, do you start picking on yourself about your weight? My girl-friend Sally, who is an actress, says when she is upset about something she automatically starts talking about her weight. When she met a guy on a blind date and he was just not a nice person, she obsessed over the experience. "He talked about himself the whole time and had a really mean kind of personality! Do you think it's because he thinks I am fat?" As she fretted about getting a callback for a voice-over commercial, she began talking about how fat she is and worried how she might not get the job. I reminded her that it was a *voice*-over, not a *body*-over commercial!

For years, my default setting was obsession about my body. It took a long time to realize that putting all my focus on my weight distracted me from dealing with other issues in my life. If you do the same, be aware of it. When you're on a rant about the size of your body parts, you need to stop and get in touch with what you're really upset about. I wonder, sometimes, if the reason so many of us who have gained weight and lost it have trouble maintaining the weight loss is that we don't truly accept ourselves, and we don't feel deserving of our new bodies. What would hap-pen if, instead of hating ourselves, we practiced radical self-compassion?

MOVEMENT: WHERE THE HECK IS THAT PART OF MY BODY?

All living creatures need to move to keep themselves healthy. Our bodies are mostly made up of fluids that have to flow through our systems. Letting your blood and lymph fluids stagnate and pool is not good for you. Also, movement prevents and limits depression, prevents panic attacks, and builds up your body's immunity, as well as your muscle strength and flexibility so that you don't strain muscles or tear ligaments when you're doing everyday activities.

Okay, I bet you're rolling your eyes now that I am about to talk about movement and exercise. You know it all by now! Everybody who has had weight issues knows about exercise, but a unique quality of people who feel too much seems to be that they lack the level of general body awareness that normal people develop from birth. They struggle with something called *proprioception*, which is how the body senses itself. When asked, "Do you know where your body is at all times?" how would you answer? Do you have to think about the answer longer than most people do?

When you close your eyes, and someone says move your right leg, proprioception is supposed to tell you where it is without your having to look down at your leg. Proprioceptive receptors for stimuli are located in the joints and ligaments, and signals are sent through the nervous system up to the brain's sensory processing center, which puts it together with other information (such as your visual sense and your sense of movement) and lets you know exactly what's going on with your body in relation to your environment. This system bypasses your thinking mind, or it's supposed to. According to a theory called *sensory integration*, which an occupational therapist named A. Jean Ayres developed in the early 1970s, some of us don't have typical sensory processing going on. Somewhere along the way, the signals get mixed up, and people with sensory processing issues actually have to think about their body's positioning. They fall off chairs, bump into people and objects, and feel as if they're sort of floating. If you don't have this problem, think about how your body feels after hours skiing or on a boat and how you feel the need to stomp around to remind it that you're back on solid ground. When you're stomping, you're giving yourself proprioceptive stimulation by crunching your joints and ligaments together, and you feel as if you're back in your body. I find that, when I'm feeling as if I'm floating, not completely attached to my body, it helps to chew gum, which gives proprioceptive stimulation because chewing compresses the joints in the jaw.

People who feel too much, even though we obsess about our weight and food, have difficulty starting exercise programs because we often don't know where our body actually is in space. I have found this to be true particularly in women with abuse backgrounds; they have mastered dissociation as a survival mechanism, finding it easier to "live in their heads." I know I have this because every time I have begun to work with a trainer, I have to concentrate 100 percent on what the trainer is telling me to do; if she says, "Move your right foot!" I might otherwise easily move my left. Hey, it's a foot—I got that part right!

It's essential for people who feel too much to start developing body awareness and acknowledge that this is an issue *before* beginning to exercise. Otherwise, you might hurt yourself. You might also become demoralized because you feel so uncoordinated. Classes in rooms with mirrors are especially hard because you have to see your body reflected back; try not to compare it to the bodies next to you, and follow the instructor's verbal directions and movements, which you can see from the back as well as in the reflection in the mirror. I have a friend who says she used to well up in tears in classes like this, until she figured out she needs to stand directly behind the instructor and mimic her moves.

MANY OPTIONS FOR MOVING

One thing that can hold people back from engaging in regular movement is emotional resistance to the idea of exercise—which is why I prefer to call it movement. Maybe you are carrying around painful memories of cruel classmates in physical education classes, rolling their eyes when they got stuck having you on the team; so many people with weight problems have that history of mistreatment. You don't have to be coordinated, be competitive, or feel miserable to get the healthy movement you need. Movement should be fun. In fact, many people who talk themselves into exercising for health reasons find that they actually end up craving that movement and go out of their way to get it; it's enjoyable and it helps them feel better, emotionally and physically.

You can also jiggle for weight release! If you're very uncomfortable with movement, owing to chronic pain and inflammation, it can be really hard to find ways to move that don't make you wince and sink into an easy chair. I know it can be frustrating to not be able to move the way you once did, or the way you wish you could, but don't give up and eliminate all movement. If movement is painful, or you are very overweight and it takes great effort to get moving, start slowly. I think whole-body vibration is a fantastic way to boost circulation, immunity, and the flow of your bodily fluids while waking up your muscles so that movement is easier. Every day, even when I'm sick or feeling lethargic, I get on my whole-body vibration machine and let the vibration go to work on my muscles, stimulating the muscle neurons and fibers to contract—more so than they would during ordinary exercising. If you've ever done an exercise that's unfamiliar or that you rarely do and thought the next day, "Wow, I can feel the burn in muscles I didn't know I had," you recognize that we tend to work with only certain muscles while others lose tone. The movement you experience on a whole-body vibration machine is low impact—you stand on a platform that oscillates—so you aren't putting undue stress on overworked, damaged, or aging joints.

Just as you would with any exercise program, you have to start slow with whole-body vibration so you don't experience fatigue and uric acid buildup in muscles, which will make them sore. Even so, it's a very gentle way to begin moving if you are out of shape. Another bonus is that it improves your bone density because the vibratory motion stimulates the cells that build bone cells while calming the cells that break them down.

Movement comes in so many enjoyable forms. Choose one that you enjoy and that's right for your body and your schedule. You can walk, swim, or do yoga, Tai Chi, or Qi Gong, none of which is too strenuous if done properly, but all of which gives a great overall body workout.

Walking is great because anyone can start doing it at any time, without special equipment—all you need is some quality, supportive walking shoes. Think about walking on a more giving surface than a floor or sidewalk to put less pressure on your joints. Try a track designed for runners, or a grass or dirt path.

If you love to swim, do it in an ocean, lake, river, or pond that you know is not too polluted. There's no such thing as a pristine body of water anymore, but find a spot to swim where you won't be exposed to too many environmental toxins. If you swim in pools, favor the ones that are kept clean without the use of harsh chemicals. I love swimming; in the summer, I make it a habit of swimming at least four times a week in a saltwater pool. I don't swim particularly fast, but I love its wonderful effects on my mind, body, and spirit. And I'll push myself a teeny bit more each time, not because I want to punish my body but because I love it and want it to be strong and healthy.

With any form of exercise, if you overdo it in order to compete with others, bullying your body as if you were in boot camp with a military officer swearing at you, you are more likely to hurt yourself, physically—and emotionally. Remember, kindness and self-compassion are your goals. Also, just because a gym advertises that it welcomes people of all body types and all levels of fitness, the people who work out there may be competitive and judgmental. Exercise in places where you feel welcome and are accepted. You don't need to take in anyone else's negative feelings when you are trying to shed your own along with the pounds!

If you enjoy vigorous, stimulating movement, and your body can handle it, by all means train for a marathon, do rigorous sports, or take a class that involves fast, exciting moves. However, don't feel this is the only way to get in the movement you need to maintain good health and keep excess weight off. According to the Centers for Disease Control, walking at a good clip, during which you are just a little out of breath, or doing a similar exercise for two and a half hours a week along with spending some time twice a week moving every muscle group, is all you need to stay healthy. Maybe you have to make a little more effort to keep your BMI under 25, or you prefer to exercise more to relieve stress or to be more fit. Other organizations have different recommendations; but frankly, the idea that you have to work out heavily for at least an hour every day, without fail, isn't in synch with your body's actual needs.

Dance to music you enjoy, in your living room if that's convenient—or make dancing a social occasion. Instead of getting together with a friend to eat out or have a drink, plan a date to try line dancing or hiking through a nature preserve. When I lived in Sedona, Arizona, my favorite Pilates instructor was a vibrant young woman named Rima, who had the best Zumba class ever. She was the most sensual, expressive dancer, and watching her at the front of the room was an experience in and of itself. I danced at the back of the room, sometimes moving in the same direction as everyone else and sometimes, well, not! Did I have fun? *Yes!* It gave me joy to watch Rima and it gave me joy to stumble around at the back of the class! It didn't have to be perfect for me to love every luscious moment of it.

Take a fitness class together with friends and encourage each other. A friend of mine was feeling uncoordinated in a class when the woman next to her whispered, "You're doing great. This is my fifth time in beginning salsa. I'm not ready to go on to the more advanced one!" Why pressure yourself? There's no physical education teacher standing over you anymore, threatening to lower your grade if you don't work harder, and there are no tests.

Another enjoyable way to get movement is to play an active video game by yourself or with friends or your kids, or just play with them outside, kicking a ball around. If you love dogs, you might get one you can walk. You'll enjoy being with your furry friend while getting much-needed movement.

Movement has an even stronger effect on our spirits and attitude when we exercise outdoors. Every day, I love to walk by the ocean near my house. "Green exercise" outside near the grass and trees combines movement with being in the sunlight, which helps us to manufacture serotonin, the feel-good hormone, and vitamin D, an important nutrient associated with less depression and irritability (as well as better immunity and less risk of dementia, among other benefits). In fact, one study shows that just five minutes outside in nature can boost your mood; and being in nature offers a host of health benefits. If you're stuck inside, surround yourself with plants and pets. As I said before, it's easier to feel peaceful and in touch with your spirituality when you're in nature under open skies, or looking at the rich array of plants, insects, and animals in a forest or alongside a river, or gazing out across the breadth of mountains, an open field, or a large lake or ocean. Walk, hike, or bike, and maybe rest or meditate when you're outdoors, too.

If you haven't biked since you were a kid, check out the bicycles that are available now. You have many choices, including reclining bikes that are low to the ground and may be more comfortable if you struggle with balance or feel clumsy. You don't have to impress anyone. Don't feel you have to push yourself to do something that takes more coordination and skill than you feel you have.

If you want to keep track of how many steps you take each day, or how many more free weight repetitions you can do to help you stay motivated, go for it. You don't have to compete with anyone else, or be hard on yourself if you don't make your goals as quickly as you thought you would, or fall behind because you became ill.

In fact, think about working with hand weights regularly to keep your muscles toned and your bones strong, and to raise your metabolism (having too many fat cells lowers your metabolism while increased muscle mass raises it). You can keep a set out where you spend a lot of time to remind yourself to use them. Lifting weights, starting with one-pound free weights and working up to heavier ones, is a great way to become more body aware, get in a little movement, and build strength—and it helps build bone density. Keep in mind that when you increase your muscle mass, it boosts your metabolism and helps you burn more calories, even at rest. Don't overdo it, though; you have to give your muscles a chance to rest. If you have poor upper body strength and build up your strength with weight lifting, even using lighter weights, you'll enjoy an added bonus of not feeling sore after carrying a heavy suitcase or packages.

I first began to train with hand weights several years ago, when I was a recording artist and was terrified of being perceived as heavy. Now, my motivation is very different. I do it for my health and overall well-being: I want to have a fit, healthy body because I love myself. It's far better to work out because you love yourself than because you're afraid someone is going to point at you and call out, "Fatty!"

Movement can also prevent the back pain brought on by poor posture. Building your trunk muscles through core exercises, yoga, and other forms of movement address these problems and make it easier for you to not feel fatigued when you have to stand or sit a lot.

Whatever movement you do, focus on strength, stamina, health, and movement; and check in with your body to be sure you are doing what's right for you. If you feel pain, stop. "No pain, no gain" should not be your mantra! You aren't trying out for the Olympics; you're working to be healthy, raise your metabolism, and manage your moods. Pain does nothing to help you achieve those goals; in fact, pain can sap your motivation (if you do overdo it, the salt baths, which contain Epsom salts, will help alleviate your sore muscles). Go slowly! If you find yourself intimidated or embarrassed for any reason, stop and figure out how you can change the experience so you keep it fun and enjoyable.

Movement should be something you look forward to, not something you dread. It should make you feel better physically and emotionally, and put you back in touch with your body in a positive way. That's especially important if you often disassociate from your body because you don't like it, or you feel it has betrayed you, or you've been a victim of physical or sexual abuse. You may never be as slim and as trim as you would like to be, but you can enjoy your body's strength, flexibility, and fitness.

Make sure you move *every* day. If you're not feeling well or you're tired, just do a few minutes' worth of movement to nurture yourself and your body. If you find it exhausting to even think about exercise, don't feel guilty. Read the next section, because you may have an underlying adrenal problem that's zapping your strength. Pushing yourself when you have adrenal fatigue will make it worse.

WHEN YOUR ADRENALS NEED A VACATION

Perimenopausal and menopausal women, and people who have experienced excessive emotional or physical stress, are especially prone to *adrenal overload*, also known as *adrenal fatigue*. This condition makes you utterly exhausted, causes a slew of system imbalances, and may lead to even more serious problems. I highly recommend Dr. Marcelle Pick's book *Are You Tired and Wired?* for learning more about this increasingly common condition. For people who feel too much, who reach for sugar and caffeine as stimulants, and who experience chronic stress from empathy overload, adrenal fatigue is a serious concern.

The two adrenal glands—little organs that are about two inches across and sit atop your kidneys—have a main job and a secondary job. Their main job is to release hormones such as cortisol and adrenaline, which set off a series of biological events that give you energy when you are in danger and need great strength and speed to "fight" or "flee" (this is called the *fight-or-flight response*). The adrenals' secondary job is to create and secrete other hormones when the glands that normally have that responsibility aren't working for some reason. For example, as a woman enters perimenopause, or as a man becomes older, the glands producing the sex hormones start to shut down, and the adrenal glands have to step in to keep the hormones balanced.

If the adrenals are working overtime handling stress responses, it's harder for them to keep up with their second job, filling in as a sex-hormone generator. Being good workers, they push themselves harder, creating and releasing more hormones. Over time, with no respite from chronic stress, they become so strained from being overworked that they start to shut down. They can't produce sufficient amounts of the hormones your body needs and the result is adrenal fatigue. You feel tired, and yet wired at times, too, because your adrenals rally here and there, then poop out ("Go team! Zzzzzzzz.").

You start to depend on sugar, caffeine, and other stimulants to keep yourself awake and alert, which, unfortunately, strains the adrenals even more. You are supposed to be resting to give your adrenals a vacation, but you can't, so you knock back a few cups of coffee and munch on a doughnut so you can keep going full speed ahead. Your hair may be thinning, you're getting fog-brained and forgetful, and headaches are plaguing you. Your sleep cycle is disrupted by insomnia and the inability to fall asleep or wake up clearheaded, and the sleep deprivation lowers your metabolism and makes it harder to lose weight. Meanwhile, all these physiological responses cause you to feel depressed, angry, and anxious, and these emotions signal to your body to keep going with its attempts to battle the stress. It's a vicious cycle.

Underlying all these symptoms are imbalances in your body caused by overworked adrenals that are either in a state of fatigue or overactive and about to burn out. For example, adrenals are responsible for preventing blood sugar fluctuations, which cause fierce cravings for sugar, dips in energy, and, eventually, diabetes. Adrenals also play a major role in a healthy immune system, and when they're overtaxed, you experience more infections, including yeast overgrowth in your gut and in the warm, moist areas of your body.

Additionally, your adrenals are responsible for making sure you maintain the right balance of fluids in your cells and your blood. When your fluids are imbalanced, you retain water, crave salt, and ache because of swollen joints or tissues. When you're experiencing all that, you're hardly ready to bounce out of bed and start your day. You move less, your metabolism slows in order to ensure that you're holding on to plenty of energy to fuel yourself, your fat cells store that energy, and you gain weight.

Fluid imbalance is also called *inflammation,* which is the precursor to a host of diseases and conditions from heart disease to autoimmune disorders. Heart disease is the number one killer of American women, and 70 to 90 percent of people with certain common autoimmune disorders are female. Women who feel too much, who put enormous energy into taking care of others at the expense of their own health and well-being, are at high risk for adrenal fatigue, inflammation, and autoimmune disorders such as fibromyalgia, diabetes, arthritis, lupus, sarcoidosis, and pulmonary fibrosis.

Did You Know ... ?

Did you know there's evidence that the prolonged stress of caretaking can lead to autoimmune disorders? Taking care of those who need help is wonderful, but when it's a detour away from managing your own porous boundaries, or causes you to develop adrenal fatigue, you have to set some boundaries and tend to your own health. If you're caretaking for your aging parents, and your siblings aren't pitching in, ask them to help take the pressure off by contributing practical or financial aid. Talk to a social worker about programs for assisting not just your parent but you as a caretaker.

In an autoimmune disorder, the body doesn't recognize its own cells and it treats them like the enemy. It's interesting that our "angry," inflamed tissues are associated with an internal battle against the very cells we are supposed to love and nurture because they are a part of us. So here we are, worried about our weight, feeling guilty and angry with ourselves, beating ourselves up for not losing the extra pounds, pushing ourselves to exercise and cut calories, and perhaps exacerbating an underlying problem of adrenal fatigue. Cease-fire! We have to use a loving, healing, compassionate approach to bringing the body back into balance, reset our metabolism, restore balance and peace of mind, and return to a healthy weight.

If you suspect you have adrenal fatigue, don't push yourself to exercise because then you can become even more wiped out. Clean up your diet; consult a medical health professional and a nutritionist to be sure you're supporting your adrenals through diet and supplements, and maybe even medication; and reduce your stress. This program will help, but don't underestimate just how much of a toll chronic stress takes on you. Taking care of yourself and managing your emotions are very difficult when you're tired and wired.

CONNECTING TO YOUR EMOTIONS AND THOUGHTS

Emotions and thoughts are very closely related, especially for people who feel too much. You can talk yourself into or out of a bad mood, for instance. It can help a lot to use cognitive therapy techniques to pick apart your thoughts and see whether they are distorted in a negative way. "I'm never going to get all my work done!" or "I'm always hungry!" may describe how you feel in the moment, but those statements aren't literally true. If you say them often enough, you'll believe them, so catch yourself when you're thinking in terms of all or nothing, "never" and "always," or when you're minimizing any evidence that you're doing well and maximizing any evidence that you're a total screwup. Catch yourself thinking negative, distorted thoughts and replace them with healthier, more supportive thoughts.

Once again, being neutral and nonreactive keeps you from being completely overcome by strong emotions. You can say to yourself, *Of course, I'm not always hungry, but I am now because I lost track of time and should have had lunch a couple of hours ago.* That sort of logical thought process can prevent you from feeding your fears, lessen your negative self-talk, and clue you in to what you need to do: plan your meals a little better and have some healthy snacks on hand so you don't ruin lunch by wolfing down a candy bar at two o'clock in the afternoon.

Thoughts and emotions drive each other. If an emotion is very strong and distressing, use the IN-Vizion Process and let your intuitive right brain show you in symbols what you are experiencing emotionally. Once you sit in the observer's chair and become neutral and nonreactive, what to do next becomes much clearer. Then your overactive mind won't jump on the horse to the land of endless, anxious inner chatter.

Negative self-talk leads to negative moods that are artificial. Are you aware of the constant chatter inside your head? What is its quality? As you work with affirmations and the EFT each day when taking your salt bath, you'll start to replace that constant babble about how awful you are with internal thoughts that support you and make you feel good. I also recommend that you use affirmations in other situations. Peggy McColl, author of *Your Destiny Switch*, suggests that every time you do something habitual, like get into your car to start it, or stand at the sink to brush your teeth, you say affirmations and believe them wholeheartedly. It's easy to think, *Yeah, I should do that* but never get around to it. Find ways to create the habit of speaking to yourself in ways that are inspiring and energizing.

CONNECTING TO THE LARGER WORLD THROUGH MEDIA

Now that you've had a break from the media and social media for several weeks, you can also start to see how that has been affecting you. If you looked back at a newspaper from two months ago and read the headlines—and I encourage you to do this!—I'll bet you'll see that, had you not been aware of the daily news, it wouldn't make one bit of difference in your life today. Most of the news we're exposed to is designed to stimulate us into staying tuned to the media outlet through the advertisements, so that we buy, buy, buy. You hear a horrible crime story that happened thousands of miles away from you, remain riveted and in a state of shock and fear, and you sit through the commercial about a gooey, yummy brownie mix ("Lower in fat! Indulge yourself! You deserve it!"). You find yourself putting on your coat to run to the store. Marketing that hooks you in with a response of fear or anger is very effective for the company that is selling you something, but it's not good for your emotional state.

Rather than going back to the old habit of devouring the daily news, think about what news you really need to stay informed and be a responsible citizen in your community and on your planet. Chances are that the news you really need doesn't trigger emotional overload for you. Listen, it might be kind of boring, but oftentimes boring is good for you. It's tempting to tune into 24-hour news channels and absorb all the live reporting on a tragedy or a drama, but it's too stimulating for people who feel too much and it doesn't make you better informed, anyway. Recently, there was a tragedy in the news and the emergency call to the police from the victim was released to the media. I knew this was the last thing I needed to hear. My heart had broken for the poor soul already. I didn't need to take in the intense anguish that I'm sure could be heard on the recording!

To balance all the negativity you hear, take in news that is uplifting, inspiring, reassuring, or energizing. Check out scientific and health breakthroughs—they're usually something to cheer about, or at the least, intriguing without being overstimulating and making you anxious or upset. Read about the positive changes that are happening in your community or around the world. If you went by the national and international news coverage only, you would swear that the only thing that ever happens in Africa is that people die from violence or starvation, even though many Africans are living very happy, productive, peaceful lives. Yes, we need to know about problems, but we also need to know about solutions. Think about ways you can limit your exposure to the negative stories and increase your awareness of all that's positive in the world. Subscribe to "good news only" news services, if you can. *The Huffington Post* now has a "Good News" section. You can also subscribe to the *Good News Network, Happy News,* and *Good Press News,* for example.

Also, if you can, read your news rather than watch it in video form or looking at photographs. Generally speaking, images are much more likely to trigger fear, anxiety, despair, and anger than are words, especially if moving images are involved. It's hard to pull your eyes away from the screen when you're watching horror unfold before you. Visual images speak to our hidden fears and our emotional center so quickly that our thinking brains are a step behind what's happening. But when you read about a tragedy, your emotions are tempered somewhat, and you can easily look away and make a conscious decision whether or not to continue reading. While there are people who are so distanced from their emotions that they need to see images of violence and suffering to have their empathy aroused, that's not your problem as a person who feels too much. You may not be able to handle images of graphic violence. That said, I have consciously chosen to watch People for the Ethical Treatment of Animals (PETA) videos on the abuse of animals in factory farms, and that triggered action on my part, so I'm glad I saw them. I've watched footage of animal cruelty because I didn't want to keep my head in the sand; I needed to educate myself on where my food came from and how the animals we eat are treated. I know it will help me stay committed to cruelty-free eating. You have to decide for yourself about whether you want to watch these disturbing images to get some benefit from the experience. Be mindful of how these images affect you, prepare yourself for the viewing, and be gentle to yourself afterward. Whatever you decide, don't become overwhelmed and start thinking that there's nothing you can do to help people and animals to avoid or to heal from trauma. Use your disgust, horror, and anger to fuel positive actions.

CONNECTING TO OTHER PEOPLE

Now that you're aware of the danger involved in soaking up every emotion in the room when you are around other people, you can remain neutral and nonreactive when you are at social gatherings, in crowds, or with people who are upset. You can visualize a slippery blue bubble around yourself and can cut any cords tying these people to you energetically. It should be easier to avoid isolation or its complementary behavior, enmeshment.

Enmeshment can creep up on us. We think we're being loving and compassionate, when we're actually being controlling and codependent; that's because we can't stand our feeling of empathy overload. We focus completely on other people and on getting them to do what we want them to do, rather than on attending to our own emotional agitation. In short, we detour away from our emotional discomfort.

Use the techniques in this book to prevent becoming overwhelmed by your emotions; but at the same time, think about practical ways you can maintain good boundaries. Don't take in the world's drama! Do you have to bring your smartphone with you everywhere you go, and check your messages instantly? Are you addicted to social media? Maybe you have developed the habit of being reactive to the world around you and need to break the addiction!

We have *so* many sources of stimulation these days, from social media, to cell phones, to constant interaction with other people (if we live and work in a highly populated area). Technology can keep us connected at all times, but it can also be used to disconnect us from others when we need a break. Use a software program to keep you off the Internet, or at least off of particular Internet sites that are addictive and that overstimulate you. Find ways to organize your incoming messages so that you don't feel the need to sort through hundreds of them to see if any are actually important. For instance, have more than one e-mail address—one for information you know is low priority and one you only use for the most important messages.

Set physical boundaries with other people, too. Maybe you need to wear earplugs or noise-cancellation headphones sometimes (just be sure you don't use them all the time or you'll get used to dead silence and have even more trouble tolerating background noise when it's unavoidable). Limit how often you talk to people who leave you exhausted after a conversation with them! Just because you love your hyperactive, needy sister, that doesn't mean you have to get into her latest drama every time she calls.

Remember, try not to share garbage with other people. Bond with others over solutions, not problems, and laughing, not complaining. If you do listen to someone sharing garbage, don't get enmeshed and try to solve his problems. Just nod, acknowledge that you're listening, and do deep, slow breathing if you feel yourself starting to take in his anger, frustration, or negativity.

If you need to vent, okay, but don't dump on other people, and put some limits on that venting. Use your Sacred Box and your Dumping Grounds journal to get the garbage out of you, and then *stop* obsessing over it. Would you pick through your kitchen garbage all day long? I don't think so! Don't obsess over the garbage that comes up for you, and keep it from contaminating your relationships with others. If you realize you've been dumping, say, "Thanks for listening and letting me share," and move on to a more positive subject. (Don't forget to do your garbage dump at the end of week two of this step.)

Finally, don't underestimate the importance of serving others from a place of strength and love, rather than a place of neediness and desperation. Giving out of a longing to have someone notice you or validate your worth is not good for you, and it's a detour away from managing your difficult emotions and from sorting through your own issues. It can be easier to be the angel of mercy and hear gushing praise for your self-sacrifice than to face your self-loathing or your shame, but detouring will burn you out and leave you fatigued and depressed. You'll just end up facing the very emotional issues you've been trying to avoid that never went away.

Serving others should leave you feeling stronger and renewed. It can be a great antidote for sitting around feeling sorry for yourself and obsessing over your weight and your body. My way of serving others includes doing intuitive readings for people. Recently, I was connecting to the energy of a man who had died of asthma. When I do this connecting, I actually feel the sensations that the person felt—it's his way of communicating the concept to me. I've had breathing problems in the past, and feeling this man's inability to inhale deeply nearly sent me into a panic. I carried on the group reading, but afterward I had to use visualization and breathing techniques to let go of the fear generated inside me when feeling that horrible sensation. So, it's important to me to use my intuitive talents to help people, but sometimes it's very wearing. I have to balance my own well-being and my own needs with helping others.

To remind myself of the power of giving to others from a place of love and security instead of fear and desperation, I often say the following version of the St. Francis of Assisi prayer to myself:

ST. FRANCIS OF ASSISI PRAYER

When you say this classic prayer, you take your focus off of yourself and any obsessions with perfection and control and place it on a healthy relationship with others (note that you can replace the word *Lord* with *Spirit,* or any other term that feels right for you):

> Lord, make me an instrument of your peace.
> Where there is hatred, let me sow love;
> where there is injury, pardon;
> where there is doubt, faith;
> where there is despair, hope;
> where there is darkness, light;
> and where there is sadness, joy.

Lord, grant that I may not so much seek
to be consoled as to console;
to be understood as to understand;
to be loved as to love.
For it is in giving that we receive;
it is in pardoning that we are pardoned;
and it is in dying that we are born to eternal life.

When you take care of others and absorb their feelings, it can be so stimulating that it's almost like taking a drug. It can even be addictive. Even after the active part of this program is over with, I hope you'll continue to deal with your discomfort in healthier ways, and prevent its recurring, by regularly using the techniques for shedding excess emotional weight.

In this week's daily journaling exercises, the focus is on reconnecting to others, to your body, to your thoughts and emotions, and to the world. As you've done before, write the answers in your journal, working on a few questions every day.

DAILY JOURNALING FOR STEP FOUR:
RECONNECT WITHOUT LOSING YOURSELF

Answer two to three questions daily until you've answered them all.

1. What types of movement have you begun to incorporate in your life? What's working for you? What type of movement isn't working for you? Why? Can you adjust it to better meet your needs?

2. What are some ways you are reconnecting to your body? How do you feel before, during, and after these activities?

3. Now that you're engaging in more movement, how are your moods? What sort of thoughts are you having about your body?

4. How does it feel to have taken such a long break from traditional and social media? Can you imagine limiting it indefinitely? What would your life be like if you did?

5. Imagine yourself having healthier boundaries with people you don't know or hardly know. How might you limit your interactions with their anger, fear, sadness, jealousy, and so on, so that you're not overwhelmed yet stay connected? Think of practical solutions here. Are there ways you could use communication technologies differently?

6. List all the specific people you would like to let go of altogether, then list any emotional, interpersonal dynamics you would like to change, such as feeling obligated to give more than the other person does.

7. Imagine the dynamic with each person differently. Could you have relationships with the same people but change the energy that characterizes your interactions? For example, you may have a difficult relationship with a friend because you lack clear boundaries and you feel she drains you. If you had a healthy boundary, or if the dynamic were different (for instance, if you stopped people pleasing), what would that look and feel like?

8. Is it hard for you to imagine maintaining a problematic relationship yet changing the dynamic? Why do you think that is? What's the roadblock?

9. Is it possible that the dynamic could change but you're afraid of or uncomfortable with how it might change? Write down as much as you can about this.

10. What people, circumstances, or relationships would you remove altogether? How does it feel to think about making the choice to end the relationship rather than try to improve it?

11. What would you want to add to your relationships to make them better?

12. Who have you become now that you've been working on this program? How are you different?

13. Once the emotional and energetic clutter is taken away and you're no longer angry and ashamed, who will you be? What will your life look like?

14. Is it possible to let go of the fear of uncertainty and stop hoarding what's familiar but painful to behold? What would that look like?

15. Is it possible to let go of taking care of others and find space on the to-do list for self-nurturing? What would that look like?

16. Do you want to step back from caretaking and find another way to spend your time or make a living, or limit the amount of caretaking you do? How might you do this?

17. How has the energy of others been affecting you as you work this program?

18. Do you see a difference between how the energy of others affected you before the program and now, and if so, what is the difference? Who has triggered you to react to them and their behavior since you began the program?

19. Are the same people, or the same types of people, triggering you that triggered you before you began the program? What do these triggering people have in common?

20. Can you imagine a way to have interactions with these types of people without getting triggered? What would it look like to spend time with them?

21. What can you do to set healthy boundaries with these people without simply isolating yourself?

22. What will your life be like if you continue to use the techniques in this book to exercise your power of choice over your thoughts and feelings?

~~~~~~

The step of reconnecting to yourself and others integrates all the ideas you've encountered. I'm not going to kid you: it won't always be easy to balance your needs and everyone else's, or to stay in touch with what you're experiencing in your body, mind, and heart. There are plenty of distractions and stressors that can knock you off the path, but now you know what to do when that happens. It's really important to develop the habit of becoming quiet and listening to your inner wisdom instead of trying to figure out what to do to make everyone happy all the time.

Step Four, Week One:
Exercises and Activities

- Be kind to yourself. (Remember KISS: kindness, IN-Vizion, salt, simplicity).
- IN-Vizion exercises as needed to help you manage your empathy overload and strong emotions.
- Morning journaling: What's your intention for today?
- 4:00 P.M. salt bath (or salt spritz, followed by a bath as soon as you can do it), during which you do use the EFT and affirmations, to speak your truth and process your feelings.
- Daily journaling: Answer about two to three questions a day and journal about your resistance, feelings, insights, and experiences.
- Do each of the exercises within the chapter.
- Follow the simple plan of eating and movement. Continue to avoid physical stimulants and mental ones (such as the news and social media).
- Evening journaling: How did you do today? What is one thing you did right? What is one thing you're grateful for?

Step Four, Week Two:
Maintenance Exercises and Activities

- Be kind to yourself. (Remember KISS: kindness, IN-Vizion, salt, simplicity).
- IN-Vizion exercises as needed to help you manage your empathy overload and strong emotions.
- Morning journaling: What's your intention for today?

- Journal daily or every few days if you find journaling helps you to sort out your feelings.
- 4:00 P.M. salt bath (or salt spritz, followed by a bath as soon as you can do it), along with EFT to process your feelings.
- Follow the simple plan of eating and movement. Continue to avoid physical stimulants and mental ones (such as the news and social media).
- Evening journaling: How did you do today? What is one thing you did right? What is one thing you're grateful for?
- End of week: Dump the garbage.

And that's it—the four-step plan! In the next chapter, I provide you with a lot of information and ideas about healthy foods, but I can't tell you exactly what to eat because I don't know your body. At this point, you're ready to start thinking about changing your eating habits permanently, and incorporating foods that are better for you because you're not nearly as likely to obsess or become anxious. Remember, you should *enjoy* eating. Let go of the negative feelings about past experiences with food and open yourself up to a new way of relating to it. The good news is that now that your emotions have been quieted, you'll probably find it's a lot easier to avoid the noisy foods that trigger disordered eating.

KEEP IN MIND . . .

- Begin reconnecting to your body. Do the I Love My Body! exercise and express love to your body regularly.
- If you find yourself obsessing about your body, ask yourself whether you're detouring away from difficult emotions about something else altogether.

- Many people who feel too much have difficulty with proprioception—that is, their sense of body awareness. If you feel clumsy and awkward, do exercises that don't take a lot of coordination and be gentle with yourself.

- People who feel too much can also have poor body awareness because they began to dissociate themselves from their bodies after suffering an assault or rape. Reconnecting with the body is very important for healing from these types of traumas.

- Consider using a whole-body vibration machine as a gentle way to start to get exercise and build body awareness, too.

- Get yourself moving in ways you find enjoyable. You may do better with low-stimulation exercises, such as walking, swimming, and yoga, rather than high-stimulation exercises such as aerobic exercise classes. Assert yourself in creating opportunities for movement that make you feel comfortable. Change instructors or classes if you have to.

- Be compassionate with yourself as you begin to get movement. Don't feel you have to push yourself. You really only have to do the equivalent of brisk walking for an hour twice a week and doing movement that works all the muscle groups twice a week, but if you really want to do a marathon, that's fine too.

- Movement can be more fun if you do it with a friend, work out to music, or get "green exercise" in nature. Research shows there are extra mood-boosting benefits to exercising outdoors. Think about biking or walking (a pedometer can help you keep track of your steps).

- Lifting hand weights builds bone and muscle mass, as well as strength, while giving you exercise. Boosting your muscle mass also boosts your metabolism.

- Whatever movement you do, focus on strength, stamina, health, and movement; check in with your body to be sure you are doing what's right for you. Forget about "no pain, no gain"—it's not true.

- Know the symptoms of adrenal fatigue and address them, getting any needed tests to check your hormone levels and reducing your stress.

- Reconnect with your feelings. Experience them, use the IN-Vizion Process if they're intense, and don't turn up the volume on them by thinking negative and distorted thoughts.
- Reconnect with your thought processes. Become aware of negative self-talk whenever it occurs and immediately replace it with positive self-talk that supports happiness and confidence.
- Reconnect with the larger world and stay informed about what's going on, but limit your exposure to bad news. Balance it by going out of your way to find good news sources.
- Avoid watching disturbing news on video or listening to the audio. Read your news instead to limit your empathetic response so you're not overwhelmed.
- As you reconnect to other people, use the techniques in this book, such as The Slick Blue Shield exercise (Chapter 4), to set boundaries, but also set healthy boundaries in practical ways, too. You don't always have to take someone's phone call or continue a relationship with him or her.
- Break your addictions to communication technology, whether it's your smartphone or social media that's making you enmeshed with others and overstimulating you. Use software programs to keep you off of social media when you're using your computer.
- Don't bond with others by dumping your garbage on them or letting them dump on you. Bond by encouraging each other.
- Beware of the detour of caretaking—the dysfunctional dynamic of codependency. Don't deplete yourself while giving to others and don't take responsibility for their emotions and choices.

PART FOUR

It's Simple,
but It's Not Easy

8

Now Let's Talk Food!

As I said before, I'm a full-on, flag-flying foodie. I love food and I love to eat, and I don't just enjoy a good meal, I savor it. I had to learn to appreciate the taste, texture, and temperature of food again after years of bulimia in my teens and early 20s, which had me using food as a mood modifier. If it was going to spike my serotonin level, fast, and quiet my anxiety, I was going to eat it. Later, when I began to be more mindful of what I was eating because I had my porous boundaries under better control, I realized that some of my trigger foods tasted awful. Now, if I'm going to have a small portion of cake, I'm going to take my time and enjoy it, without the accompanying cacophony of thoughts around how "bad-bad-bad" I am for eating it. Deprivation has never worked for me, nor for any of my students; and one of the most important pieces I have learned is that if I say I can't have it, I will want it—for the wrong reasons.

As I began to make peace with myself, my body, and my life, I found I could choose to have a small piece of cake once in a while without its sending me off to the store to buy a whole cake, devouring it on the way home! *Restoring the ability to make choices is crucial.* If it's a crappy, rock-hard, processed "treat" out of a package, blechh! And, if it's a food that is generally noisy for me, I avoid it altogether. I don't want to even contemplate a box of cookies, as they are likely going to be singing, "Eat me, eat me!" once I have the first one. I have no desire to do that to myself anymore. I know what works and I know what doesn't; I'm very clear that tempting myself with a trigger food is an incredibly bad idea. As an ex-addict and recovered alcoholic, I know that a glass of wine isn't okay for me, either. Certain foods just don't work for me. And so what? There are plenty of other delicious choices that will make me feel good and healthy, rather than compulsive and crazy! *When you no longer feel compelled to manage your empathy overload by grounding yourself with food, making good decisions about what to eat is infinitely easier. When you stop beating up on yourself, you'll notice your triggers and learn how to avoid them.*

What should you eat? When I decided to write this book, it was because I had discovered a link between empathy overload and weight issues. That's what I'd experienced, as had a large portion of my clients. So, this was never meant to be a typical diet book, which is why we don't talk about food until now. Everyone is different. For example, people have different blood types and unique genetics, so different bodies can respond differently to the same food.

As I always advise my students in my online classes, visit a nutritionist or health coach, see a doctor, get blood work done, find out your hormone levels if you're middle-aged, and learn whether you have any vitamin or mineral deficiencies. These are things I can't address.

EATING WHAT FEELS RIGHT

Food plans are personal, so I'll share what works for me and give you my general advice on eating for people who feel too much. In short, what I recommend is pretty basic: try to consume a predominantly locally grown, plant-based diet, as free as possible from chemicals and environmental toxins. Limit consumption of stimulants, especially if they are noisy foods for you. Stay away from processed foods, and avoid all genetically modified foods; no one really knows their long-term effects, and why should you gamble? Beyond that, listen to your body's response to what are seemingly listed as healthy foods, whether they are whole-grain bread or soy products. I have a friend who wanted to add soy to her diet, but she realized that after eating a meal with a large serving of tempeh or tofu, she would get an odd headache and her stomach wouldn't feel quite right. Her body was telling her to limit soy and find another protein source.

Some of you may do just fine with small amounts of gluten in your diet, mostly in the form of whole grains, and even be able to eat white-flour pasta on occasion without gaining weight or having digestive problems, blood sugar fluctuations, or food cravings afterward. The problem is that people who feel too much also tend to be oblivious to just how much sugar, gluten, refined flour, processed foods, and chemically altered fats they are eating, the emotional distraction they provide, and these foods' effects on the body. Take gluten, for example. Did you know that gluten is added to a full range of foods, from salad dressings to ketchup to teriyaki sauce? If you cut out all gluten, you might discover you feel much better—plenty of people just don't digest gluten well. In fact, you might find you have celiac disease, which is the inability to digest gluten; you can take a blood test to determine if this is the case. So, why overload your system with something it has trouble working with, taking valuable energy away from your body's other systems? It's interesting that gluten intolerance and celiac disease have become more common since food producers started adding gluten to more foods and since growers began using genetically modified grains. Is that a coincidence?

You may find that your body doesn't handle certain foods well, which shouldn't be a problem because you have plenty of options. That said, there is just one more important factor I want you to consider when choosing foods: whether they are cruelty-free.

CRUELTY-FREE FOODS

People who feel too much are often able to pick up on the emotions of animals because those emotions have been infused in the animals' milk, eggs, and flesh. If an animal has lived a stressful, unnatural life, its very cells are affected as a result. When you take those cells into your body by eating cheese, eggs, or meat, you are actually eating their fear, anxiety, anger, and sadness, energetically speaking. Every fearful experience and mistreatment they have in their unnatural lives is an energy that is experienced and floods their systems with chemicals that are present in what we eat. Animals feel their feelings and no one who has ever cared for one can deny that. Animals can experience emotions, not necessarily in response to actual thoughts, as we do—a cow isn't having an existential crisis about the meaning of life. But the animal *is* terribly stressed and afraid by being packed into an unnaturally crowded pen, unable to wander freely under rainy and sunny skies, unable to eat a variety of grasses, and unable to interact with other species.

In North America, we have huge stockyards of cattle that never place their hooves upon the grass or drink from streams, and that eat a combination of corn and ground-up animal parts, which they would never do in nature. They are also given antibiotics to prevent and treat infections that they have developed as a result of this unhealthy and unnatural experience, and also from application of hormones such as bovine growth hormone (BGH) to enhance a cow's milk production. You, of course, ingest those antibiotics when you drink the cow's milk or eat the flesh of an animal that has been treated with them.

And it's not just cattle that are treated inhumanely; chickens and pigs, too, see such treatment. In fact, chickens' beaks, which are meant to peck the ground and help fertilize the soil, are cut off so that they won't harm each other when the crowded conditions under which they live cause them to attack their coop mates. It hurts to even think about the suffering of these poor creatures.

While animals may not seem to have the same range and complexity of emotional experience that we do, they certainly feel sadness, anger, and contentment. An animal that has no quality of life, that isn't living in harmony with the land and with other creatures, is not a happy animal. Consider what neuropeptides get into a human body when a person eats the egg of a chicken that's been caged every moment of its life, or the flesh of a fish that can barely swim in the filthy pond water of a fish farm.

If you do eat meat, poultry, fish, eggs, or milk products, think about how the animals have lived and died—peacefully or violently? Were they treated with respect or disrespect? Was that animal's life on the farm similar to the life it would have led in nature?

I can't cite any specific scientific research on the emotional effects of eating cruelty-free foods vs. factory-farmed foods; it's something I know from years of working with highly intuitive, sensitive, and empathic people. As I grew more in tune with my body, after years of abusing it and ignoring its messages, I started to recognize that eating meat or dairy products just didn't feel right. I typically buy certain brands of organic goat and sheep cheese because I know the animals are treated well on the farms that supply the milk for these dairy products; but one day, I was in a pinch and bought an unfamiliar brand of Cheddar cheese to go with my lunch. I was chatting away as I was eating, and everything seemed fine, until I started to clear my plate. Suddenly I had an overwhelming sense of sadness and panic that lasted a few moments. I knew deep down that it was because I had been eating something from a factory farm. I believe the body knows what it needs, and although I had been pretty strict "veggies only" for years, I have found that sometimes I feel much better adding some grass-fed free-range beef to my diet. One thing is for certain: I feel the difference between a naturally raised cow and one from a factory farm.

Even if you think it's not going to affect you when you have a burger made from a stockyard animal that has been mistreated, hear me out. Modern farming methods that treat animals as commodities instead of sentient beings are cruel and unnatural. Yet research shows that people would rather deny that an animal they eat has suffered than change their eating habits. Please don't underestimate how beneficial it is to yourself, to the animals, and to the planet to eat a mostly plant-based diet and to consume only cruelty-free dairy, poultry, fish, and meats—if you consume animal products at all.

Educate yourself on how the animals bred for food are treated, and then choose what to do. There is no excuse for any of us to not know where our food comes from, in what manner it is delivered, and how the animals we eat are treated. We are all responsible for this planet, as well as every living thing on it. You don't have to be as extreme as I am in my commitment to eat humanely. After I read the books and watched the DVDs that are listed at the end of this book, which forced me to look at the cruelty and truth of slaughterhouses, factory farms, and dairy farms, as well as read the studies about the emotional lives of farm animals, I made up my mind. You may feel differently after learning about the origins of your food.

Also, there have been several excellent books and documentaries explaining why corporate farming is so detrimental, not just to the animals but also to the planet and to us. What producers are doing to the food we put in our bodies is horrifying. You may have heard of additives like "pink slime" (the unappetizing, informal name for the ammonia-treated beef by-products that are added to beef as a filler) or "meat glue" (the equally unappetizing name for a powder mixed with meat scraps and used to "glue together" larger pieces of meat, making it more likely for bacteria to grow in an undercooked steak). You owe it to yourself to know what you are eating. I encourage you to look at the Recommended Reading and Resources section of this book to learn more about what you are putting in your body and the ways you can eat more cleanly and healthfully.

WHAT YOU DON'T KNOW ABOUT PROTEIN

If you are worried about getting enough protein, don't be. Humans aren't designed to live on large quantities of meat, eggs, milk, and cheese. When it comes to how our ancestors ate, you probably have an image of cavemen hunting the woolly mammoth and a tribe of hunters feasting on the flesh, with a few berries served on the side. In reality, most of the calories those hunter-and-gatherer tribes consumed came from plants, and successful hunts were relatively rare. It was the women, picking berries and digging up roots, who kept the tribe from starving. (Funny how history doesn't give them credit for keeping early humans alive, isn't it?)

Somehow, along the way, we got the impression that we wouldn't be strong and healthy unless we ate plenty of meat and dairy foods. This myth of our large protein need was picked up by producers and advertisers, who make money by promoting certain products. You might be surprised to know that most North Americans eat more protein than they need. That's not my opinion; that's straight from the Centers for Disease Control. Two cups of cooked dried beans and 8 ounces of milk or yogurt will about do it for meeting an adult's daily intake of protein. That said, we do need protein in our diets so you will have to find it somehow and your particular food plan may include more of it than someone else's. When I am particularly active, I consume more protein and feel good with 100 grams per day; when I am less active, I may consume 60 grams per day. It's an individual choice.

What we aren't getting enough of is fiber and vegetables (for the record, no, ketchup doesn't count as a vegetable, regardless of what bureaucrats or lobbyists for the fast-food industry have claimed). Cruelty-free dairy products or meats may cost more, but since we don't need to eat large amounts of protein, it makes sense to spend our grocery dollars on quality protein that comes to our plate without wreaking destruction and creating fear, anger, and sorrow along the way.

Again, I'm not saying you have to be a vegan or need to boycott all meat. You may find that your body and spirit can tolerate some animal products and even feel better when you eat small amounts of them. I'd been mostly a vegetarian for years, but after a time my body was clearly craving a different protein source, so I added fish and eggs; then once I began more strenuous exercise, and due to hormonal changes, my body steered me to add small amounts of red meat back into my diet. I was very conscious about these choices and checked in with my own health care team. I believe as long as they aren't farmed in a way that abuses the animals, I can choose to eat them according to my body's needs. Moderation is the key as there is no one-size-fits-all food plan for everyone.

Whenever I buy eggs, I make sure they come from local farmers whose chickens are allowed to walk about the farmyard. Labels can be misleading. It's appalling, but some farmers restrict chickens to a tiny area outside, where they are similarly packed in, then label the eggs as "free range" and "cage free." Don't assume that every egg distributor using those labels is being totally honest. If you have any doubts about how animals on a particular farm are treated, check it out; look up the farm on the Internet. If you see "free farmed" on the label, that means the American Humane Society has checked out the conditions and has granted this certification. Educate yourself. People who feel too much are most adversely affected by cruelly slaughtered and unnaturally raised food source animals.

PRACTICE AHIMSA

The idea that growing and harvesting food should *not* involve hurting any person or animal isn't new or original, that's for sure! Hindus, Buddhists, and Jainists embrace *ahimsa*—the belief that it's important to "do no harm," including violence, to living beings. Some interpret ahimsa as meaning that you should be careful not to hurt insects, and some would simply say that you shouldn't harm or kill sentient beings and should also never harm the whole (the environment). If spraying harsh chemicals to kill insects in your home would affect living beings and the environment those beings exist in, then, according to ahimsa, you should find a better way to get the insects back into a more convenient environment, like your backyard! Frankly, those insects probably have important work to do outside, whether it's breaking down plants or dead animals, or serving as supper for songbirds.

Regardless of your ethical or religious beliefs, as a human being, your respect of this idea of ahimsa just makes sense. You share the planet with 7 billion other people and countless creatures, insects, microbes, and plants. The more the population increases, the greater the possibility that nature can't easily break down the toxins created by technology and the more we will all have to live sustainably, aware of our effects on everyone and everything in our unified world. Mother Nature cleans her waters, air, and land, but these days she can't keep up with the nasty garbage we dump on her. She doesn't even know what most of it is. Look at all those multisyllabic words on the back of a package of processed food; do you think your body, where all these chemicals will end up, has any idea what to do with butylated hydroxytoluene (BHT) and propyl gallate (two common preservatives)? And what do these chemicals do when they combine with the other foods we eat, the air we breathe, and the environmental toxins we breathe in or drink (for instance, the Bisphenol A, or BPA, that we ingest when drinking from plastic bottles or eating foods stored in cans or plastic)? What happens to this chemical soup when it leaves your body and enters the water system, and then, through evaporation of water, settles in the air and soil?

Consider the possibility of vegetarianism or veganism, if that seems to be in alignment with your body's needs. Please think about practicing ahimsa and consciously choosing cruelty-free eating. Try it just for a short time, and notice how different you feel.

HUNTING, FISHING, AND FARMING WITH RESPECT

I acknowledge that people who have grown up on, or live on, farms, or who hunt or fish, have a different relationship to animals than I have. I respect the hunter or fisherman who is awed by the beauty of the doe, pheasant, or trout before he respectfully kills it, prepares it, and uses its flesh to feed his family, even though I could never do that. It makes sense that people who spend large amounts of time in nature get to know these creatures and their habits, and they don't see them as objects to be killed, processed, and eaten. In many cases, they may be the modern equivalent of the indigenous peoples who lived on the land, who killed an animal and gave thanks to its spirit for sacrificing its body to nourish them as part of the cycle of life.

As we become more conscious of the suffering of animals, I think we'll start to see a return to farming the old-fashioned and more sustainable way, keeping the animals on the land interacting with other species and allowing their manure to fertilize a variety of indigenous plants and grains. When we took the animals off of the land, the crops suffered, too; they began to experience many diseases and were more vulnerable to pests. *Monoculture* (growing plants of just one species instead of many), which farmers do to maximize profits, has also played a role in making grains less hardy. To address this problem, many farmers learned to dust their crops with powerful chemicals that killed pests and warded off blight and fungi. Then, genetically modified seeds were introduced as a solution as well. Are conditions such as celiac disease and gluten intolerance part of the price we are paying for disrespecting and harming nature and the earth?

Life is not all about profits. We should support people who grow varied crops and heirloom produce. These older varieties of plants and animals are rare now because they didn't contribute well to a corporate farm's bottom line. Nature intended the earth to be filled with a variety of plants and animals. When we violate nature's diversity through monoculture, we set ourselves up for that limited species to be wiped out, as well as likely doing something to the balance of nature that we will regret. For example, scientists in Britain and France have recently discovered that a common pesticide is killing off much of the pollinating bee population, which is a crucial link in the food chain. If you buy organic produce, you protect those bees and all our other plants, as well as the animals and our planet.

When you practice ahimsa and cruelty-free eating, you support farmers who are not destroying the land, air, and water or harming animals. After all, those huge stockyards of corn-eating cattle pollute the ozone layer with the methane in their flatulence, their urine forms toxic ponds, and their antibiotic-laden manure can't be used to fertilize crops or even prairie grass. Creating these situations is cruel to the earth, its creatures, and ourselves. That's why I feel strongly that we should eat organic plant foods grown in ways that respect the planet and its inhabitants—including us!

We also should avoid foods that have been contaminated by antibiotics and hormones, which are now present in eggs and milk, as well as meat. Is it a coincidence that American girls are entering puberty before age 10, even as young as 6, when we have so many hormone-disrupter chemicals in our environment? All animals have flora in their guts and microbes on their bodies; we're supposed to live in harmony with these tiny plants and animals. But because we have overused antibiotics, we have created an imbalance in nature, and now we have nasty bacteria that don't respond to any antibiotics and can be deadly. When you choose foods that don't upset the balance of nature, you're eating in a cruelty-free way that respects nature and all her creatures, including yourself.

WHAT TO EAT

GOOD PROTEIN CHOICES

If you're willing to give up beef, pork, fish, dairy, and other animal products, or at the very least cut down on them and eat only cruelty-free versions, you will still have many choices for protein. Meat and dairy provide complete essential amino acids (the building blocks of protein), but you can get these amino acids by combining legumes or beans with whole grains. Quinoa, an ancient grain, is a great choice for most people; it offers a complete protein and has several minerals; because it's a fibrous grain, it contributes to colon health and stable blood sugar, just as other fibrous grains do. Quinoa cooks up in 15 minutes and has a marvelous texture and nutty taste.

Soy, which you can get in the form of tofu, soy milk, miso, soy flour, and edamame beans, is another source of protein. You can also find protein in chickpeas, chickpea flour, pea protein powder, whey protein powder, and similar products. Soy supports bone health and prevents hot flashes in women going through perimenopause. Just be sure to avoid soy isolate and TVP, or textured vegetable protein. Both are highly processed.

On the other hand, "to soy or not to soy" can be a real issue for some people. My fitness trainer vehemently says that all soy is poison, while my hormone specialist says it's okay for me to eat it! I feel fine after consuming soy, so it's part of my diet. If you do choose to eat soy, always make sure it is non-GMO (genetically modified organisms, such as bacteria and fungi, that have been tinkered with in order to provide some sort of benefit, such as a heartier grain crop). If the package says "certified organic non-GMO," then you can buy it. Edamame beans are green soy beans in their natural state and are a great low-calorie snack, as well as a protein in your salad. This is why I recommend you see a doctor and a nutritionist and get on a food plan that works for you. Not all foods are tolerated by all people. There is no such thing as a one-size-fits-all food plan.

Here's a list of cruelty-free protein foods that include legumes plus seeds, nuts, or grains:

- almond, cashew, sunflower, or peanut butter on whole-grain bread or pita
- beans or lentils with buckwheat noodles (soba noodles) or rice pasta
- handful of nuts (go for the nonroasted, nonsalted versions, which are healthier—you might sprinkle them on a salad or chop them up and throw them on a vegetable dish)
- lentil, bean, or split pea soup with whole-grain crackers
- corn or whole wheat tortillas with beans (be careful not to buy traditional refried beans that have lard, which is animal fat)
- rice and beans
- beans on toast
- hummus and whole wheat crackers or bread
- corn and beans
- veggie burgers that contain soy

Some of these foods are incredibly easy to prepare. What's simpler than breaking up some whole-grain crackers and dipping them in hummus, or spreading almond butter on a slice of multigrain bread? If you're sensitive to gluten, you can try soy and quinoa, which don't have gluten, because they have whole proteins. Alternatively, you can pair beans, seeds, or nuts with corn, rice, or, if you can tolerate it, millet (ask your doctor if that will work for you). You might be able to tolerate oatmeal, too, which you can eat with almond milk.

FRESH, SEASONAL, LOCAL, ORGANIC PRODUCE

Whenever possible, the fruits and vegetables you eat should be fresh, seasonal, locally grown, and organic.

Fresh and Seasonal

Just-picked vegetables and fruits are absolutely delicious and they pack the greatest nutritional punch. Unfortunately, we can't always have the ones we would like, given the time of year and where we live. Many of us have gotten spoiled by red grapes and strawberries from Chile in winter and bright red tomatoes on the vine in early spring, but these are far from local. Try to buy your fruits and vegetables in season, or buy them frozen, because the produce is picked at the height of the season. Often, you'll have to sacrifice the texture, because freezing and thawing can make corn, berries, and other produce mushy, but frozen is better than canned. Canned vegetables tend to be packed in water with a lot of processed salt, plus there's usually Bisphenol A in the can lining, which is no good for you.

Organic

Organic produce can cost twice as much as nonorganic produce, which is a problem for people on a tight budget. Still, I think it's better to eat quality fruits and vegetables, even if you end up having to eat less food overall. You can also choose to buy organic versions of the produce most likely to be laden with pesticides and nonorganic versions of produce that has fewer pesticides. See the following for which produce is likely to have the highest concentration of pesticides.

High-Pesticide Produce (try to buy organic versions)

Celery

Spinach

Red bell peppers

Potatoes

Lettuce

Collard greens
Kale
Strawberries
Peaches
Apples
Blueberries, domestically grown
Grapes, imported
Nectarines, imported

Lower Pesticide Produce
(again, try to buy organic versions anyway)
Onions
Eggplants
Sweet potatoes
Sweet corn
Sweet peas
Avocados
Cabbages
Asparagus
Kiwi
Mangos
Watermelons
Pineapples
Cantaloupes, domestically grown

HIGH-FIBER, FILLING FRUITS AND VEGETABLES

High-fiber fruits and vegetables are tasty and nutritious, and they also fill you up more than low-fiber foods do. Try cruciferous vegetables, such as broccoli, broccoli rabe, cauliflower, kohlrabi, Brussels sprouts, cabbage, collard greens, kale, bok choy (Chinese cabbage), turnip, rutabaga, and radishes. For fruits, eat raspberries, blackberries, pears, apples, strawberries, bananas, and oranges.

SEASONINGS AND CONDIMENTS

Many of us grew up reaching for processed salt, ground black pepper, ketchup, mayonnaise, butter or margarine, and bottled salad dressings to make our food taste better. One thing you'll notice as you start buying fresher, organic, local, in-season produce is that it's far more delicious and the taste is much more intense than you might expect; you won't feel the need to drown it in butter or salt! It's fine to use condiments, but think about fresh herbs, healthier oils, lemon juice, and homemade salad dressings—or at least, bottled ones that don't contain chemicals and fillers like gluten.

For healthier oils to use on your food and in cooking, avoid anything heavily processed, such as palm kernel oil and anything made from genetically modified corn or soybean oil (that eliminates all canola oils, as well as many name-brand oils you'll find at the grocery store). Use extra-virgin oils that are organic and expeller pressed. I recommend extra-virgin olive oil, which is high in omega-3 fatty acids. My favorite brand is Lucini, but there are many terrific ones, especially from Portugal and Greece. I also recommend organic extra-virgin coconut oil, which is high in saturated fats but when used in moderation is very good for you compared to other fats. In the morning, I can spread a little coconut oil on a piece of Ezekiel bread and I'm full for hours.

Many processed foods lose flavor in the processing, so a lot of extra salt is added and then we shake processed salt on to them to give them even more flavor. Instead, give up the processed foods and salts, and avoid kosher sea salt, which is becoming more processed, and more polluted, than ever before. Salt from the Dead Sea has been touted as having health benefits, but studies show it has a lot of toxins. Table salt, even kosher sea salt, is heated, causing the natural crystals to break up and become irregular, and precious minerals are destroyed in the process. Buy a salt grinder and use Himalayan salt on your food instead. Take a bag of it with you when you're traveling or going to eat at a restaurant.

Many spices not only bring flavor to your food but are also incredibly healthy for you. Turmeric (also found in cumin and curry) is an anti-inflammatory and is also good for digestion and for boosting the immune system; it's an appetite suppressant as well. Turmeric may also help prevent Alzheimer's disease as well as cancer, so eat your curry! Cloves are good for alleviating arthritis, fungal infections, bad bacteria, and infections. Cinnamon helps treat arthritis pain and also helps lower bad cholesterol, keep blood sugar levels stable, and boost cognitive function and memory. Garlic lowers cholesterol levels and is good for your heart. Cardamom contributes to healthy circulation and digestion. Marjoram promotes good digestion, as does fennel, which also helps reduce gas, works as an appetite suppressant, and helps reduce the amount of bone loss suffered after menopause. Ginger can relieve headaches and menstrual cramps, along with arthritis pain and nausea. Jamaican allspice is good for your digestion and helps you maintain healthy blood sugar levels. Oregano is an antifungal that can kill yeast overgrowth and fungal infections. Cayenne pepper helps your body clear itself of toxins and contributes to good circulation. Sage helps reduce inflammation, so it can help ease arthritis pain.

If you love soy sauce, you might want to replace it with Bragg's amino acids, which has a very similar taste and texture but is free from added salts and GMOs.

HEALTHIER SUGARS

After working through the four steps of this weight-loss program, you have come to realize that you've been using—and abusing!—sugar as a way to ground yourself and avoid painful or overwhelming feelings. Now that you have some healthier alternatives, think about taking most or—drum roll, please—*all* the sugars out of your diet. People who feel too much need to avoid high-glycemic-index foods, and sweeteners are at the top of that list. A spike in blood sugar is like an invitation to detour away from yourself quicker than you can say "candy-coated rocket ship"!

Personally, I avoid white sugar as much as possible. If I use a sweetener, it's rare, but it will be either a teeny bit of dark organic agave or real dark amber Canadian maple syrup. Stevia is an option, too. Sugars are present in fruits and vegetables, but if you eat them in their raw form, or cooked but with plenty of the fiber preserved, they won't wreak havoc on your system. It's the fruit juices you need to be more concerned about. If you have strong mood swings or symptoms of low blood sugar (hypoglycemia), be extra cautious about consuming sugar. There is a brilliant video one of my certified coaches posted on our special Facebook Weight Release Energetix coaching page, called "Sugar: The Bitter Truth." It's long, but I highly suggest everyone watch it. All my coaches must watch this video, and they also must encourage their clients to watch it.

Did you know that the University of California has a video series on the subject of sugar and how it hurts our bodies and minds? To view it on YouTube, go to: http://www.youtube.com /watch?v=dBnniua6-oM&feature=em-share_video_user.

This is a very interesting and informative series with Dr. Robert H. Lustig, "The Skinny on Obesity," at http://www .uctv.tv/skinny-on-obesity. Dr. Lustig is professor of pediatrics in the Division of Endocrinology at the University of California, San Francisco. He explores the damage caused by sugary foods, arguing that fructose (too much) and fiber (not enough) appear to be cornerstones of the obesity epidemic because of their effects on insulin.

GRAINS

Not everyone can handle the gluten that's present in most grains, but if you can tolerate gluten, whole grains can be a healthy part of your diet. Read the food labels carefully: "Made from whole grain" doesn't mean that the food necessarily *contains* whole grains. All grains start out as whole grains; it's what is done in the processing that leaves them without fiber! (How misleading are some of these food labels? It's really annoying!) Go for brown rice instead of white rice; white rice is missing the hull. Buy whole-grain breads and pastas, not ones made from refined flours and dyed with a bit of molasses to make them look healthy! If you're avoiding gluten, you've got options, such as brown rice pasta.

WATER

It's important to stay hydrated. Most experts agree that thirst is a good indicator of whether you need more water, so you probably don't have to measure exactly how much you're drinking. The water in fruits and vegetables counts as your water intake, but you'll also need to drink water to be sure you don't become dehydrated. When you aren't eating a meal or snacking, drink ionized water to keep your body as alkaline as possible. When you're having water and eating at the same time, put a slice of lemon in the water. It not only gives the water a little flavor but it increases the water's alkalinity, which reduces the acidity in the body. I use an ionizer at home and drink alkaline water as much as possible. You will have to decide for yourself whether you think alkaline water is important, but whatever you choose, make sure you stay hydrated, particularly on hot days and when you're getting movement.

WHERE TO FIND GOOD FOOD

FARMERS' MARKETS

Do an Internet search to locate farmers' markets in your area. Not all farmers' markets are open year-round, but when they are open, they offer super-fresh produce. Of course, you'll probably also find booths selling candy or cookies or other treats, so be aware that noisy foods may call to you while you're checking out the leafy greens.

One thing I've found is that the produce sellers are often eager to let you have a taste and to educate you on how to store and cook a vegetable or herb that's unfamiliar to you. You start to become familiar with which vegetables and fruits are in season. In-season produce tastes the best and is more nutritious. It also tends to last longer in your refrigerator because it hasn't had to travel a long way. Local produce can go from field to your table on the same day. If you haven't had just-picked vegetables or fruits, you really have to try them.

Time your visit to farmers' markets carefully. The most popular fruits and vegetables, or the ones that are at the end of their season, can sell out quickly. The best deals are at the end of the day. If you're making soup, you might pick up a big bag of marked-down produce the farmer doesn't want to drag back home.

FARMERS' COOPERATIVES

In some areas, you can contract with local farmers to receive a weekly shipment of whatever fruits and vegetables are in season. You may be invited to help harvest the produce as a way to keep your costs low, or you can to go to a specific location to pick up that week's boxes of vegetables and fruits. If you choose this route, be forewarned that you may end up with large amounts of a vegetable you don't like or have no idea how to prepare. You have to be ready to learn how to cook seasonally—and think about trading some of that huge bag of zucchinis with a friend.

URBAN FARMS

Vegetables and fruits can be grown in empty lots, in buildings under artificial light, or atop skyscrapers in cities. These are urban farms. There's hope that urban agriculture will radically change the food landscape, making it easier for city dwellers to obtain local, organic produce. One of the advantages of growing foods indoors is that it's a way to extend the growing season. Another is that animal waste, such as the water that fish live in and excrete in, can be used to fertilize plants, while the plant waste can be used to feed the fish, resulting in both healthier plants and animals. It's also easier to avoid using pesticides and antibiotics, and to grow foods organically, when they aren't sharing air space with pesticide-laden crops in the field across the road.

Similarly, urban farmers are discovering that, with the right types of greenhouses, or vertical farms within buildings, they can grow produce in the bitter cold of winter because the crops are sheltered from the weather. These methods are likely to open up many more options for people living in those "food deserts," where grocery stores are rare and produce isn't fresh or of high quality. By supporting organic farming and urban agriculture, you're being both friendly to the earth and a good citizen. Check to see if there are urban farms near you. If they don't sell directly to consumers, they may sell to your local food co-operative or health food store.

Did You Know...?

Refrigerators today aren't the energy hogs they used to be. You might want to think about trading in your old refrigerator for one that uses as little as one-third of the energy used by an older, inefficient model. Also, if you get a model with the vegetable drawers on the side or in the top compartment, rather than at the bottom, you may end up eating more vegetables. That is, when you have to bend over or sit on the floor to go through the vegetable drawer, it's easy to talk yourself into buying takeout instead of seeing what produce you have on hand!

HEALTH FOOD STORES AND CO-OPS

Some grocery stores specialize in offering healthful foods instead of highly processed foods. Their prices may seem high compared to the same foods at the standard grocery store, but there are reasons for this. First, many of the items are organic and it costs more to grow and distribute organic foods. Second, smaller companies may not be able to offer the large discounts that standard stores get. Third, processed foods are often less expensive because they are loaded with cheap fillers, such as high fructose corn syrup, and have chemical preservatives that keep them from spoiling on the shelf. That's convenient for the grocer and keeps his losses low, but it's not good for your body, which has to process all that junk. One aisle to head toward is the bulk aisle, where you can find rice, whole grains, peanut butter, and other staples in larger quantities. Selling these items in bulk can keep the price very reasonable. Be sure to pay attention to when you bought these items, and store them carefully so they don't spoil in your cupboard.

Some health food grocery stores are co-ops owned by the people who shop there. At some of these co-ops, you simply buy a membership; others require that you spend a few hours a month working there. Look into your local options.

GROCERY STORES

Learn where the healthiest foods are found in your local grocery store. Usually, they're somewhere on the edge of the store, in the produce aisle. Pay attention to sales flyers because the produce on sale is probably what's in season. Over time, you will get to know when it is the best time to buy your favorite fruits and vegetables.

Healthy fruits and vegetables can often be found in the frozen food aisle, too. Frozen food is picked and quick-frozen at the height of its freshness, so the taste and nutrition are optimal. However, if you're particular about textures, you may prefer to buy fresh produce, since freezing can render your corn soft and your strawberries mushy. You can always use the frozen versions in soup, stir-fries, or smoothies, where the texture is going to be altered anyway.

Some grocery stores have an aisle devoted to packaged health foods, from cereals to pastas, soups, and more. However, you might find that no particular food source has everything you want. Maybe you find the best produce at the farmers' market in the summertime and the health food co-op in the winter, and you fill in with foods from the grocery store. In time, you'll get to know which places have the best selection and prices.

That said, make a point of not going to the grocery store when you are hungry, angry, lonely, or tired—think "HALT!" In these emotional states, you're likely to find yourself buying comfort foods you don't want to bring home. Even a health food store or a farmers' market can have a tempting aisle or stall. Have you ever found yourself standing in front of the wholesale bins of grains, dried fruit, and cereals, salivating at the conveniently placed bin of your favorite binge foods and fantasizing about getting them home and hiding them in some secret spot so you wouldn't be caught bingeing on them? Be mindful when you shop and always remember that food shouldn't be entertainment. Linger as long as you like in front of the Brussels sprouts and those cute purple carrots, though. You're unlikely to start plotting a way to consume them in massive quantities, as you would the one-bite "healthy" brownies, carob-covered peanuts, or the cookies made from all-natural ingredients.

YOUR GARDEN

Growing some of your own food can be fun and easy, even if you don't have a backyard. You can rent a plot from a farmer, neighbor, or your community (one of my clients rents a plot at the local elementary school). You can also create beds on your urban rooftop or plant in patio containers. One of my students lives in an apartment and plants all kinds of veggies and herbs on her balcony, saving herself hundreds of dollars.

Growing at least some of your own food is gentle to the earth. You can save food scraps for composting, which cuts down on the amount of garbage the sanitation workers have to cart away from your home. Also, produce shipped from far away uses up a lot of fossil foods in transport, so gardening reduces your carbon footprint. In fact, in America during World War II, the government encouraged people to plant "Victory Gardens" in their backyards, so that the precious resource of gasoline, needed to move troops and equipment, wasn't used to truck produce all over the United States. We have fewer family farms now, but we still have backyards and porches and empty lots.

Go to a gardening center and ask a lot of questions about which crops grow best where you live. They will help you learn about soil, mulching, staking your tomatoes or other climbers, and how to keep the critters out of your garden. Talk to your neighbors about what vegetables and herbs grow well for them. You can start with seeds, but you don't have to—pick up seedlings at gardening centers and farmers' markets to give you a good start.

And although you might roll your eyes right now, loving your plants, playing calm and beautiful music when you plant the seedlings, even praying for them, creates happy, healthy, good-for-you food! Research shows there is such a thing as bio communication between all life-forms. Remember the experiment I mentioned in Chapter 2 described in Lynne McTaggart's book *The Intention Experiment?* It seems logical that being loving and kind to the plants you eat would have a positive effect on them, too.

Author Denise Linn and her amazing chef-daughter Meadow Linn have a beautiful, inspiring book called *The Mystic Cookbook* that is becoming a classic on conscious eating and the sacred connection we have with the food we eat. It has some delicious recipes that are so good, perfect for people who feel too much, and includes suggestions on beautiful sacred rituals and prayers for food.

OBSERVING WHAT YOU EAT AND WHY YOU EAT IT

Did you know that keeping a food journal has proved effective in helping people lose weight? You might want to create such a journal on paper or online (many websites offer you the option). In the journal, you record *everything* you eat, including portion sizes and condiments, for a few days or a couple of weeks; this gives insights into what you are eating, how much you are eating, and if and when you are eating in a disordered way. Then you can journal about the patterns you've noticed.

For example, do you nibble mindlessly just because food is in front of you? If your bank has cookies and coffee in the lobby or the receptionist at work has a candy jar, be conscious of that and make a point of not indulging. Does your journal reveal that you are overeating in the evening and eating very little for lunch and in the afternoon? It's harder for your body to process food effectively late at night, so eat your meals and snacks long before you go to bed.

Often, people who feel too much also obsess about food and eating, so don't use a food journal for more than a week if you find yourself constantly thinking about snacks, calories, and whether you are eating too much. Be very aware of the detour of perfectionism; don't let your food journal become an excuse for focusing all your attention on food and avoiding dealing with your feelings. I would rather you journal about the emotional experiences of eating. That said, when I knew I had to write everything down, I was less inclined to put things in my mouth unconsciously.

Mindfulness is what we're aiming for. Are you eating what you are hungry for, or are you skipping the step of tuning in to your physical and emotional needs before lifting up your fork? What is your relationship with noisy foods? Are you constantly creating dramas around them? Can you imagine a way you could "eat just one" and not think about it anymore, or can you imagine not even wanting to eat even one chip or cookie and no longer thinking about it? What's stopping you from saying no to noisy foods? What foods do you crave, and why do you think that is?

Some food cravings have a physical component. Blood sugar fluctuations can cause you to crave sugar, and adrenal fatigue can cause you to crave salt. Hormonal imbalances can cause cravings, and eating too many fats can make you crave more fats. Your brain's pleasure centers are triggered by certain foods, particularly sweet, fatty foods, so any memories of feeling good while consuming certain foods can exacerbate cravings. If you felt good not just because the cake felt pleasurable in your mouth but also because eating it made you feel grounded, or because cake reminds you of the birthday cakes your mother used to make for your special day, that only makes it harder to resist a physical craving for the sweet-fat-carbohydrate combination in cake. If you reduce your stress, stay on top of your hormone levels (particularly after adolescence, giving birth, or going into menopause), and avoid foods that you know will trigger disordered eating, you'll have an easier time controlling your cravings.

SOCIAL PRESSURES THAT AFFECT YOUR FOOD CHOICES

Sharing meals is part of our emotional heritage as human beings. We are not meant to eat alone, yet shame can drive us to eat privately in order to avoid having others comment on our eating. Isolating ourselves to avoid empathy overload can drive us to eat by ourselves most of the time, too. As I said before, eating in front of a television is a habit, and it's associated with being obese, probably because when you're focused on what you're seeing on the screen, you're not focusing on what you eat.

In the past, you may have been shamed by others because of how you ate. Maybe you were ridiculed for being a picky eater, or for overeating, or for insisting on separating foods from each other so they didn't touch (this is a common behavior among people very sensitive to food textures). Maybe you didn't like the traditional foods you were served at home, and were told you were being inauthentic for not appreciating Mom's cooking. If you left behind your social class or your ethnic neighborhood and began eating around people with different traditions and practices, you may be embarrassed by what your tastes are, or feel pressured to eat as your friends do instead of how you would like to eat.

Journal about these experiences. How often did they happen? How likely is it that people you would eat with today will criticize you the way Grandma or your father did? Are you carrying over old hurts into new situations and assuming that eating alone is the only way to avoid being scrutinized for what you eat and how much you eat?

Most of us have experienced social pressure to eat a certain way, or to eat particular foods when we didn't like them. If you were a member of the "clean plate club" and your mother expected you to eat everything you were served—and she doled out the portions—you learned not to be in touch with your own hunger and tastes. My mother insisted I eat until I saw the roses on the china plates, no matter if I liked the food or not. To this day, I cringe when I see an antique plate with a multiple rose pattern!

It can take time to relearn how to listen to your own body when eating. Remember to check into what you are hungry for before you sit down to a meal or a snack, as described in Chapter 3. If you are going to eat with others and are afraid they're going to judge you, set boundaries with them. Make your weight and eating habits subjects that are off-limits to them so that you can enjoy meals with others without feeling you have to defend yourself or sneak off to eat the way you'd like to eat.

NUTRITION AND HEALTH

I could write an entire book on how nutritious it is to eat a plant-based diet with healthy oils and sugars (such as real maple syrup or the sugars in whole fruit), in moderation. You can help prevent cancer, heart disease, high blood pressure, and other diseases and conditions by eating well. I don't think it's the best idea to obsess over fiber counts, antioxidants, minerals, and so on. If you focus on micronutrients, you'll go crazy and get confused by food packaging. I've seen cereal boxes with labels like "No fat or cholesterol!" Well, of course, it doesn't have fat or cholesterol. No grain does. What it won't say is "Ridiculously low fiber content and preservatives!" They're not going to brag about that.

The more nutritious the food you eat, the healthier you will be. You'll feel better and look better. You might start noticing that your hair, skin, and nails look more vibrant, or that you have more physical stamina. Maybe you'll be less irritable or anxious now that you rarely have to run to the bathroom because of a digestive problem and your mild heartburn has gone away. Of course, if you have a specific condition, such as an autoimmune disorder or asthma, there may be specific foods you have to avoid. For instance, the foods in the nightshade family—such as potatoes and tomatoes—can trigger flare-ups of arthritis, but you may be able to get away with different versions of certain foods (such as plum tomatoes). Listen to your body and notice when you're not feeling right. Think about what you've eaten that might have triggered the response. There are so many healthful foods that even if there are some you can't enjoy, there are plenty you can.

And, of course, I suggest getting some tests done for your unique profile to find out what supplements you need to best support your overall well-being. One of my Master-certified Weight Release Energetix coaches, Dianne Solano, is also a specialist in *orthomolecular nutrition*. That's the science of how nutrients interact with our genes to help turn on or off messages of health and disease. All living species have survived on nutrients since the beginning of time; however, we have unprecedented evidence that human health has been deteriorating over the years, owing to nutrient-poor food production and environmental toxicity. Orthomolecular nutrition restores optimal amounts of nutrients through the practice of proper food choices and supplementation to provide the best cell environment for optimal health.

Science has proved that what you eat directly affects how you think and feel. The most energy-dependent system in the body is the brain. Studies show that a day of intense concentration and emotional stress is equivalent to running a marathon, and this intense firing of brain neurons can leave us in a state of depletion. People who feel too much are especially prone to this form of exhaustion. Lowered food-nutrient status and emotional, physical stress has left us in a deficit, resulting in impaired cognitive function, sleep disturbances, weight gain, anxiety, depression, and other imbalances. Brain function, stress, and your emotions are a whole-body phenomenon.

Orthomolecular nutrition is an approach to creating a healthy mind and body. It's no longer about counting calories; it's about nutrient density. Dianne's suggestions are well documented by others in the medical profession. For people who feel too much, these supplements work especially well in conjunction with this program. Of course, see your doctor before taking any supplements.

THE TOP FOUR SUPPLEMENT RECOMMENDATIONS FOR WEIGHT LOSS AND EMPATHY OVERLOAD

The goal of providing this list is to simultaneously promote health, weight loss, and cognitive function:

1. **EPH/DHA Omega-3 Essential Oils** Unlike omega-6 and omega-9, omega-3 is the least available in our food supply. Its direct link to weight loss is as follows:
   - increases protein building by 20 percent; more muscle means faster metabolism
   - balances hormones resulting in a more balanced physiological response
   - is considered "brain food," as it helps with mood and cognitive function

   Always buy top-quality of this supplement. Fish accumulate toxins in their fat tissues, also known as bioconcentration. Look for products that are third-party certified assayed pure.

2. **Dehydrated Plant Nutrients** Critical for their amazing ability to maintain proper pH, these promote alkalinity in the body, as we all naturally tend to be acidic. All hormones and enzymes are very pH dependent, and the research is starting to show that some bodies may need double the amount of a hormone at a new pH set point. As such, there is a big link to imbalanced hormone activity, such as thyroid function; this is a key player when it comes to weight and health imbalances.

3. **Probiotics** These friendly bacteria offset the bad bacteria that circulate in all our systems. Fungi and yeast like *Candida* pose a real threat to overall health and energy. If these microorganisms exist systemically in high numbers, your cravings for sugar and carbs go up significantly.

4. **L-carnitine** Amino acid that has a direct link to fat burning.

CALMING NUTRIENTS AND HERBS

- **Saint-John's-wort**—An herb that usually comes in tincture form and can increase the amount of the neurotransmitter serotonin. Helps with anxiety, sleep challenges, or depression.
- **Kava kava**—The root of a plant that potentiates "Gaba," a neurotransmitter in the brain that gives you a sense of relaxation and calming. It is available as a powder, tea leaves, or tincture.

- **Magnesium**—Eighty percent of overall body processes use magnesium; therefore people can have a deficiency. Magnesium is great for muscle contraction; it also provides a soothing, calming effect. Magnesium can also aid in proper bowel function, as it supports strong muscle contractions, thus reducing the body's burden and toxicity—a direct benefit to weight loss and alleviating other health challenges.
- **Camomile tea**—A flowering plant prepared as a tea can help with sleep and relaxation. Known as a calming, anti-inflammatory, and antimicrobial agent.

HEALTH FOODS TO SNACK ON

When we are in emotional overload, we can teach ourselves new health-promoting habits, as opposed to sticking to old patterns that no longer serve our physiological state. These new snacking habits can include:

- **Raw nuts and seeds**—Give you the crunch if you are anxious and feeling too much and you just want to put something of substance into your body. In a raw state, nuts and seeds can be very health-promoting, as they are nutritionally complete, made up of protein, carbohydrate, and good fats.
- **Healthy dips**—Soothing to the soul and health promoting, dips can be tasty and fun. Go with what you like, but keep it clean. Choose fresh veggies such as zucchini, broccoli, celery, carrots, or sweet peppers, as opposed to chips. And remember, the more color, the better when it comes to veggies. Dips to try and store in your fridge include hummus, guacamole, and tahini.
- **Nut bars**—Easy to find and store at home, or take with you when on the go.
- **Protein shake ice cream**—It takes a little creativity, but I discovered this years ago when I wanted something like ice cream but healthy. Prepare your favorite protein shake, add some fresh berries, and place in the freezer for about 20 minutes.

You'll be surprised at how the cold and the texture make it feel
sinful—but it's not!

WHEN BUYING FOOD: THREE TOP INGREDIENTS TO STAY AWAY FROM

High fructose corn syrup
Artificial sweeteners: sucralose, aspartame, saccharin
Hydrogenated and partially hydrogenated oils

AND DON'T FORGET THE ADRENALS

Under moments of perceived stress and high emotion, these glands kick
in to do the job known as the fight-or-flight response. Earlier in the book,
I discussed how this response plays a big role in why people who feel
too much can gain weight so quickly, as well as have the hardest time
releasing it. The adrenal glands produce the stress hormones that enable
you to get away from perceived danger. A response that was critical to
human survival many years ago now causes us problems. Human life-
styles have changed so much, especially in the last hundred years, but we
continue to respond to emotional situations or even phone calls in the
exact same way as our cavemen ancestors. Eek, rhino alert!

This situation presents a typical syndrome for those of us who are on
empathy overload, as it can eventually leave us in a state of depletion
where we start to feel constant symptoms of lethargy and fatigue. Many
people suffer from adrenal exhaustion, yet it is not commonly diagnosed
in the conventional medical health model. Therefore, many people live
lives in which they are considered "healthy" by medical standards, yet
they feel that something is just not right. You can find various "Adrenal
Dysfunction Score Quizzes" online that can give you an indication of
your severity. You can also get some in-depth testing performed, such as
checking your blood serum DHEA level via a blood test or your cortisol
levels through a saliva test.

To learn more about adrenal fatigue, read James L. Wilson's book

Adrenal Fatigue: The 21st Century Stress Syndrome, which is a comprehensive, easy-to-read review of this subject that particularly plagues people who feel too much.

Adrenal Support Products

The following products help build your resiliency to stress and help you better adapt to the issues in your life caused by an empathetic nature.

Asian ginseng—A traditional Chinese root that helps the body cope better with mental, physical, and emotional stress. It is known as an *adaptogen,* as it helps lower stress and raise energy levels.

Rhodiola root extract—A root extract known as an energy booster, this helps with mental energy, alertness, and performance because it can influence levels of neuropeptides, like endorphins. Helps with mental drain and fogginess.

Cordyceps—An exotic mushroom that also acts like an adaptogen by alleviating feelings of lethargy and regulating blood pressure. It increases oxygenation and ATP production at the cellular level, resulting in more energy.

Bacopa—An herb that is great for treating a stress response that leaves you feeling anxious and jittery. It plays a protective role regarding the synaptic nerves located in the brain, thereby improving brain function and memory under stress.

Vitamin C—Although vitamin C is a great antioxidant that has many health benefits, it is taken up by the adrenals in very large amounts. You'll want to be generous with this vitamin during times of stress and emotional fatigue.

Black licorice—This is a root (not the candy) that usually comes packed in black syrup and is great for low blood pressure and dizziness resulting from adrenal exhaustion.

Helps add stamina and energy. If you suffer from high blood
pressure or fluid retention, you need to stay away from this,
however.

DHEA supplements—A low-dose hormone that your body
produces, DHEA supplements can help regulate your immune system and help build up the adrenal gland if you are
experiencing a feeling of burnout.

MEAL PLANNING AND COOKING

It takes more time to cook than to eat out, but it saves you money and
keeps you from being tempted by dessert trays. If you're pressed for time,
try recipes that take very little time to prepare. Also, you can always
make a big batch of something on a day when you have extra time, such
as during a weekend, and either freeze some of it so you aren't eating
vegetarian chili for lunch and dinner four days in a row or trade with
a friend who would love a batch of chili after four days of eating lentil
soup. In some cities, you can even find services that bring you fresh,
home-cooked meals prepared with high-quality local ingredients or that
allow you to assemble meals to take home to use the same day or freeze.

So what can you prepare if you're short on time and money?

Salad

If you store greens carefully, and use a salad spinner to dry them, you
can make up a big salad that will last for a few meals so you're not constantly making a salad from scratch. Mix it up. I often start with several
types of greens, lemon juice, herbs, and Himalayan salt, then add any of
the following:

- fresh, organic, raw corn kernels
- nuts and seeds
- seed sprouts (especially pumpkin seeds), which contain enzymes
  that help with digestion

- shrimp or tuna for some protein, or perhaps some parmesan cheese
- daikon radishes
- jicama
- cabbage

You can also add mushrooms, carrots, green pepper, red bell pepper, celery, and other vegetables to create a variety of shapes, textures, colors, and flavors.

I also like to shred baby kale, then add lemon, garlic, olive oil, and organic parmesan cheese, then let it stand for 30 minutes before eating it. The olive oil softens the kale and makes it chewy.

I've seen several cute containers for carrying a salad and separate dressing as an on-the-go meal—it's easier than ever to make salads a regular part of your diet.

Simple Vegetable Dishes

You can sauté spinach in a little oil and garlic, then add almond slivers for a simple vegetable dish. You can also sauté squash, onions, and red and yellow peppers in olive oil and garlic, or prepare grilled vegetables, laying them on the grill or spearing them with kebob spears.

Bean and Lentil Dishes

Three-bean or lentil salad, refried beans (without lard, and preferably homemade), chili, and lentil or bean soup are good options for getting cruelty-free, healthy protein. If you're pressed for time, remember that lentils cook more quickly than other beans or legumes do, and you can always keep some canned, organic beans on hand if you're in a rush. Do the best you can and try to find beans and other typically canned foods packaged in glass containers instead, as they have no BPAs.

Raw Foods

Chopping up fresh raw vegetables to dip in hummus or bean dip or to throw into a salad doesn't take a lot of time. You can pay extra for a crudités and dip tray at the supermarket, but the vegetables probably won't be consistently fresh, or organic, and the dips are often filled with ingredients you can't pronounce. Buy a sharp knife and a cutting board, and spend a few minutes chopping, or throw big chunks of vegetables into a food processor to chop or julienne (slicing them into thin strips). It's time-consuming to peel and chop, but while you're playing prep cook, you can share the chore with your partner, roommate, or kids and use the time spent preparing a meal to talk together.

Popcorn

Popcorn is a nutritious, inexpensive, whole-grain snack. I like to air-pop it and season it with Himalayan salt and olive oil. Keep in mind that corn is one of the vegetables along with soy that is most commonly genetically modified, so always look for "certified organic" or "non-GMO," or the word *heirloom* right on the package, and your body will be able to digest the corn.

Preserves

Buy fruits or vegetables in season and learn to can or preserve them. You can even do this in a city apartment, using produce from a nearby farm when the fruit is at the height of its freshness.

Juicing

I love to juice. Most people are familiar with fruit smoothies made in a blender, but these contain a lot of sugar and can make a person with hypoglycemia (low blood sugar) light-headed if not eaten with a little protein and fiber (try some popcorn and a small piece of cheese on the side). I like to make smoothies with a carrot or celery base. One of my favorites mixes carrot, celery, kale, spinach, and ginger. Invest in a quality juicer because I think you'll use it a lot once you realize how convenient it is to whip up a healthy juice drink.

Soups

Try lentil soup, split pea soup (it's great with rosemary added), or vegetable soup, and add beans for protein. For stock, keep the rough spots you cut off of vegetables—the end of the carrot or celery, for instance—in a container in the freezer until you're ready to throw them in some water on the stove to make stock. If you soak beans, use the excess water as stock. You can also buy stock to use as a base; just be sure to buy stock that doesn't have MSG, loads of processed salt, and who knows what other additives.

For soup making, a slow cooker is a great tool. You can put all the ingredients in it before you leave for work and come back with your main dish ready to go. I don't always have time to cook the way I like to, so my slow cooker has become my best friend! All you have to do is throw in the ingredients and let it simmer for a delicious, healthy happy meal!

Sandwiches

Sandwiches don't necessarily require big slices of bread. You can make an open-faced sandwich using a whole-grain, high-fiber bread or make a wrap using a tortilla (if you're avoiding gluten, use a corn tortilla).

Vegetable Dishes as Main Courses

Make a Chinese stir-fry in a wok and throw in some tofu, beans, or nuts to give it some protein. Raw, steamed, and sautéed vegetables don't have to be relegated to a tiny portion of your plate. Make them the focus and have a small portion of protein on the side.

Dip and Crackers or Pita Slices

Bean dip, fresh guacamole, and salsa (avoid the sugary ones made from mango, pineapple, etc.) go great with whole-grain crackers or pita slices, as well as raw vegetables.

Whatever you eat, remember that it should support your body, your emotions, and your spirit. Now that you know these aspects of yourself (along with your thoughts) are always intertwined, I think you'll better understand why it's so important to eat cruelty-free food that is produced in ways that sustain the earth, and to avoid the foods that will send you back into the old habits of detouring and grounding with sweets and treats instead of managing your porous boundaries.

KEEP IN MIND . . .

- Eat a predominantly locally grown plant-based diet, as free as possible from chemicals and environmental toxins.
- Limit stimulants, especially if they are noisy foods for you.
- Avoid processed foods (including soy isolate and textured vegetable protein or TVP) and genetically modified foods.
- When choosing foods, listen to your body's wisdom about what you can tolerate.
- Consider cutting out all sweets, processed flour, and gluten.
- Think hard about eating animal products. If you feel they're right for you, eat cruelty-free versions.
- Don't skimp on the protein, and use quality protein sources such as beans, seeds, nuts, soy, and whole grains like quinoa, as well as cheese if you're not avoiding animal products. And remember to choose cruelty-free meats if you are eating animal products.
- Try to eat fresh, seasonal, locally grown, organic produce. If you can't afford organic produce, focus on buying the organic versions of the dozen or so fruits and vegetables most likely to be doused in pesticides.
- Eat more high-fiber fruits and vegetables, which fill you up and are good for your system.
- Use better-quality condiments, such as Himalayan sea salt.
- Use healthier sugars, such as stevia, agave, and maple syrup, but be careful not to overuse them if sugar is a noisy food for you.
- If you eat grains, go for whole grains. Read labels carefully. "Multigrain" is not the same as "whole grain," which retains its fiber.
- Stay hydrated. Consider drinking alkalinized water or water with a slice of lemon as your usual beverage.
- Look for healthy foods at farmers' markets, farmers' cooperatives, urban farms, and health food stores and co-ops. Healthy, organic produce and meats can sometimes be found in a grocer's frozen food aisle.

- Think about gardening so you can grow your own food, even if your garden is made up of a few containers on your porch.
- Observe your eating patterns and any social pressure you might feel about eating or not eating certain foods. Journal about your observations.
- If you want to eat nutritionally, don't obsess over micronutrients. Just follow the simple rule of eating a mostly plant-based, organic diet.
- Plan meals and snacks, and cook ahead. Your options include salads, bean and lentil dishes, raw foods, popcorns, preserves, juices or smoothies, soups, sandwiches, vegetable dishes, and dips with dipping crackers or vegetables. Think about what you can eat, not what you can't eat!

Challenging Situations for People Who Feel Too Much

As I'm sure you have experienced, the best of intentions fall away when you are under stress or are distracted. When I was writing this book, I was in the midst of many major changes in my career and my life, menopause and thyroid issues not the least of them, and it was a huge challenge to process my emotions and avoid the detour of grounding through food. One thing I've learned is that there are always times when we simply have to do our best, and make peace with ourselves and our lives in the present moment. Progress, not perfection, is always my motto.

That said, you will be better prepared for challenging times by understanding what it is that makes them so stressful and distracting, and having practical strategies you can use to get through those times more easily and avoid detours and disordered eating. Let's look at situations that are common triggers for sliding back into the old behaviors and losing control of your porous boundaries, and what to do about them.

WHEN YOU ARE CELEBRATING

The simple acts of breaking bread to bond with others, treating yourself to a small indulgence, or expressing love or appreciation to someone you care about have inspired a massive global industry of producing and selling junk food. Advertisements tell us to celebrate with a particular wine, beer, or Champagne, or give ourselves a break from cooking by serving the family some carbohydrate-laden pizza-like substance that gets popped into a microwave. *Pick up convenient packages of cookies and candies "for the holidays"! Stock up on tortilla chips and soda pop for the big annual sports event! Save money buying a "family pack" of sausages to grill when you celebrate Independence Day!* And that's just the American merchandising of junk food. All around the world, food packagers have caught on to the money to be made with the "special holiday edition" of some traditional treat, infused with preservatives and processed oils to extend the shelf life. Trust me, your grandmother would not recognize the ingredients on the label of that food advertised as "just like Grandma made."

Even if you don't come across advertisements to indulge in noisy foods, you'll be reminded of their existence when you go to the grocery store. There's an entire science of retailing that dictates the placement of junk food: it's no accident that it can be found at eye level in spots where shoppers linger, such as the end of an aisle or at the checkout. Cheap, processed food can be found around the globe now, even in India, where obesity and Type 2 diabetes rates are soaring. It is very hard not to be bombarded with messages urging you to "treat yourself" with cheap junk food.

Indulge yourself, express your affection, and make occasions special— but find a way to do it that doesn't involve noisy foods and disordered eating. If you're celebrating on your own—maybe treating yourself for sticking to your intentions to manage your porous boundaries and your disordered eating, or for getting through a rough day, think about non-caloric treats. Buy some flowers, a music CD, or a book instead of candy. Let yourself watch junk TV or your favorite movie or old shows that you've seen again and again, or play video games or online games.

If you want to celebrate with others and make it special, give the gift of time: help them to set up or clean up after a party, or hang out on the porch with them watching the sunset and having a conversation. It might sound hokey, but really, don't you find that when you do spend time just enjoying the people you care about, you actually feel better afterward than if you had all sat around a big table stuffing your faces all afternoon?

What if you have to spend holidays or large gatherings with strangers? Does the social anxiety or just the dread of taking in all that emotional stimulation make you want to hide out in the kitchen, nibbling? If the celebration will include foods you don't want to eat, and Mom will insist that you try just a little of the birthday cake, have a plan for what you are going to do to deal with the emotional pressure. You do *not* have to take a mouthful of high-fat, high-salt, high-sugar, highly processed foods ("Just try one—it can't hurt!") to please other people. I know it can be hard. Keep in mind that sometimes the pressure is coming from someone who herself wants to limit sweets and alcohol but doesn't feel she can, and doesn't want to be the only one eating and drinking too much. If you think about it, you probably know someone like this. Her discomfort with your eating rules is hers, not yours, so don't take it on.

Even if you are having a great time socializing and not feeling pressured to eat nonstop, you can become easily overstimulated by the emotional pressures and start to think, *What the heck, those cookies look so cute!* or *It's only once a year that I have nachos and real cola.* It may seem as if you're just "loosening up," but you're really reaching for a quick fix for your overstimulation. This is the time to go out on the porch, tour the garden, take a walk, or find some excuse to get away from the gathering for a short respite. I know all about this firsthand, and I can list the names of all my food buddies whom I can rely on to have experienced this very situation many times. Sometimes, you do have to get away from the social pressures before reconnecting. If you are temporarily isolating yourself, and you plan to rejoin the celebration, that's fine. It all boils down to mindful choices rather than mindless ones.

I'm all for enjoying yourself and letting go of restrictions that hold you back from having a great time, but if you are really honest with yourself, actually eating that food is rarely as satisfying in reality as it is in your mind. Biting into a hot dog or a huge pile of stuffing with gravy? Is that truly delicious, or do you talk yourself into believing it is? "Loosening up" needs to be redefined. Loosen up by having fun, laughing, and moving—whether that's going for a family hike, dancing, or playing games. Loosen up by not fixating on your problems, or all the awful news in the world. When you are new to the concept of feeling too much as it relates to food and are beginning a program like this, it's important to minimize the stress from the outside, so I am not saying to ignore the things that are painful in the world—just deal with what's in front of you for now. You're learning a new skill set.

Even if you have a healthy attitude toward holidays and what to expect from them, the people around you may have a lot of emotional baggage they open up at these times and have expectations that are unrealistic. Uncle Fred is not going to turn away from the ball game and ask his adult nieces deep questions about what's happening in their lives. The teenagers are not going to automatically take their personal music players out of their ears to start up a conversation with you about how all the interesting things they are learning at school. Your alcoholic in-law is going to knock back too many cocktails and grow increasingly sullen. And, yes, your overweight, busybody aunt is going to show up with ten dozen gooey deserts that you just have to try. You don't have to be psychic to know what the plots and subplots of your family gathering will be!

Being empathic, you're likely to pick up on everyone's muddle of feelings—discomfort, resentment, shame, irritation, and frustration included. Then you'll feel a strong urge to ground with food and run around making everyone happy. And, even if you don't turn to the food, you may gain weight anyway, as your body begins to be inflamed in response to the stress. I have a student in one of the online classes of my Weight Loss for People Who Feel Too Much program who told me she will gain 8 pounds over a family weekend from stress, then lose it a few days later without even changing her food. Has that happened to you? I bet it has.

Don't get dragged into that toxic complaint corner, hoping to quiet everyone's agitation. You know the place. There's one at every gathering—the spot where everyone's standing around bitching, hissing, gossiping, and downing handfuls of junk food in big bowls. "When is he going to get himself to A.A.?" "He couldn't care less about us!" "What is *wrong* with these kids? I know we weren't like that!" *Take your hand out of the chips bowl and get away from there!*

Fortunately, there are many things you can do to manage the pressure of attending holiday and social gatherings that tend to overwhelm you.

CUT THE GATHERING SHORT OR SKIP IT

You don't want to be antisocial and isolate yourself so much that you have difficulty maintaining relationships, but you don't have to go to every gathering and stay from the moment it starts to the moment it ends no matter how grueling it gets, either. Make an excuse that you have to go to another party, and go straight home if you are too uncomfortable to admit you aren't up for a seven-hour holiday extravaganza.

Just as eating needs to have a beginning, middle, and end, social gatherings need to have boundaries if you're going to avoid empathy overload. Benjamin Franklin wrote, "Fish and visitors stink in three days." Set some limits on how much time you spend in the challenging environment of a social gathering or a family vacation. Eventually it will get much easier as you learn the particulars of self care for people who feel too much.

HAVE A PLAN FOR LEAVING

If you feel ungrounded at a social gathering, have a plan for leaving, even if only for a short time. Go to another room and do a grounding exercise (bring your saltwater spritz with you!). Offer to be the one to go to pick up your cousin at the airport 30 minutes away, then listen to calming music in your car during your mini escape. Arrange for your own reliable transportation to and from the gathering. If your family or friends can overstimulate you or upset you, you don't want to get stuck waiting for your chatty friend or relative to drive you home when she gets around to it.

START NEW TRADITIONS FOR FOODS

Bring a dish or two that you know you can eat. Make a healthier version of a traditional food. And if you want to have some control over the food and the guest list, but you're too anxious to host the party yourself, have it catered, or hold it in a restaurant or club.

START NEW TRADITIONS

Food should not be the entertainment. Host the gathering yourself or arrange with the host to get the food out of the way when everyone sits down to talk or watch the game on television. It may sound radical to your friends or family, but where is it written that you can't enjoy a gathering without constantly munching? Get everyone exercising, whether it's a walk in nature or a competition using an active video game that has everyone moving, singing, dancing, and laughing. Play a party game, whether it's charades, cards, an active video game, or a game that comes in a box. Do crafts together, or do group singing of holiday songs or funny songs everyone knows from childhood.

It's hard to snack when you're singing. If your tradition is to go to the movie theater together after your meal, avoid buying popcorn, candy, and drinks just because "it's tradition" and "it's a holiday." (By the way, movie popcorn is unbelievably bad for you. They use unhealthy oils and douse the stuff in processed salt to get you to buy a soda pop to wash it down.)

STEER THE CONVERSATION AWAY
FROM HOT TOPICS

Everyone seems to want to talk about the formerly forbidden subjects of religion and politics these days, and to voice their strong opinions. These topics can lead to tension and arguments—which is why our parents and grandparents said, "Avoid talking about religion and politics!" On top of that, there are subjects that families and groups of friends don't seem to handle well for whatever reason, whether it's competitive sports teams or personal topics such as who is gaining weight, who had an affair years ago, whose son is having trouble in school, and whose child is clearly a genius.

Don't kid yourself: you can't control all these people and get them to behave themselves and avoid hot topics, especially once the alcoholic drinks begin to flow and inhibitions get lowered. You might prepare for a very long family party by thinking ahead of time about some subjects you can introduce into the conversation. Pick some topics that are usually pretty safe territory. Go out of your way to see a new movie, catch the latest viral video, or read an interesting and noncontroversial news article that you can bring up. If you tend to be anxious, a little preparation for a party involving hours of talking can be a good idea.

KEEP IT LIGHT

If the people around you want to bring up intense, emotional subjects, you can take a break or leave, but you can also scoot out of the room and take with you some of the people who want to avoid the big argument over who said what fifteen years ago, or which political party is superior. You can also choose to smile a lot and disengage by seeing this badly written melodrama for what it is: a bit of absurd theater. Compare it to a funny movie or television show and try to predict what the next line or scene will be, and congratulate yourself for picking up on the predictability of it all. Imagine everyone as six inches tall and squeaking out their lines. Turn them into animated cartoon characters and give them funny names. Imagine famous comic actors or comedians playing their parts. Your ex-husband's lines will be much more amusing than if you took them seriously.

In short, find the craziness in the people, the situation, and the conversation and laugh inwardly. Let your mind run wild with images that make you giggle. Maybe your squabbling sisters should just have a cat-fight you could turn into a viral video and make a fortune off of—I'm not saying you should actually *do* this, but it's much more fun to fantasize about that than trying to referee their latest passive-aggressive duel over who got more attention growing up.

Humor is a powerful tool for managing your tendency to be reactive. It empowers you because humor is based on the truth, and people who feel too much often avoid the truth because it's too painful—either their own emotions, such as anxiety or embarrassment, or the emotions of others, which they take in, make them uncomfortable. Become the Laughter Goddess. Banish the storms with a belly laugh.

Of course, some people will grumble and bristle if you make light of some serious topic they want to discuss. They thrive on conflict and negative attention, and if that means they have to pick a fight over the proper way to make guacamole, damn it, they're going to have their drama! If there's someone in the group who can manage to stir up anger, anxiety, and tension no matter what the topic, physically avoid him and switch the subject, crack a joke, or walk away as soon as he delivers the opening line to his emotional drama. And let him make the guacamole his way.

No matter what, people who feel too much need to remember this motto: life is short so leave the drama at the door! Drama is exhausting and life-draining and rarely solves anything when you get dragged into it. All it does is feed the other person's self-centeredness and self-righteousness (because the other person always seems to cast herself in the role of the poor, hard done-by martyr or victim, doesn't she?). If you join in, the person feels great and you feel like crap. Do you have people in your life like this? Be careful. The anxiety these relationships trigger will not be worth it in the end.

Long-standing friends and family members who exhibit these signs feed the compulsive need that people who feel too much have for helping and rescuing. Your boundaries become so enmeshed that you feel caught in a web of confusion, and you will have a very hard time maintaining your equilibrium. If you are the one who creates the drama, then consider if drama is one of your detours. Family gatherings and holidays bring this trait out with gusto. Stay grounded. Stay centered. Stay sane.

ANNIVERSARIES OF LOSSES

The time of the year when someone you loved passed, or you were a victim of a crime and lost your sense of innocence and sense of security, can make you especially sensitive. When a loss is fresh, you expect to feel sad as the anniversary approaches, but as time goes on, you might not realize how much these anniversaries continue to stir up old pain. You might find yourself irritable and sensitive all day long, then go to write out a check and instantly recognize the date and its significance.

Holidays are often emotional times because of all the reasons I explained above, but also because they can remind us of what we lost—the dream of a marriage that lasts forever, or of a perpetually happy and healthy family. It's as if our painful experiences are held like fossils in amber. Every year, regardless of how I have changed and how much my husband loves Christmas, I can still hear the echoes of Christmases past reminding me of a dreaded holiday of drunken arguments and the feelings of fear and loss hanging in the air between my parents. I know that in time, these memories will fade in intensity as they're replaced by happier memories of my being with Marc and our two "furry children."

If you're like most people who can feel too much, you can start to obsess about the past and pull yourself, and others, down into sadness—or friends or relatives can try to drag you into their depressive attitude. Holidays tend to inspire fantasies of perfection anyway. Maybe it's because advertisers are great at pumping out images of blissfully joyful people gathering together in harmony as they open their presents from the big department store that's having a holiday supersale. Then again, maybe marketers are just responding to our own habit of thinking that whatever problems are present in our relationships, they'll magically disappear for one day or one holiday weekend and we can reclaim the old fantasy.

I lost both my parents, in different years, around the holidays. Both of them became terminally ill around Thanksgiving and died the following February. Even though it has been a very long time since I had those experiences, I know—and expect—that I will be more sensitive and open to other people's feelings during that holiday season. Emotional triggers for me are everywhere, and I'm extra careful to do my self-nurturing work so that I don't start detouring into disordered eating.

Take a few minutes to identify the times of year when you have experienced significant losses. Have you found that you're more emotional, more prone to detouring at those times? Journal about your experiences, and remember the next time those dates roll around why it's more of a struggle to manage your porous boundaries and avoid emotional overload. Just being aware of these triggering times can help you minimize their impact on you. Then, too, as I said before, *plan* for being more sensitive. Maybe on that significant day, you need to take some time off from work or chores to do something that lifts your spirits, or maybe you want to spend more time meditating or journaling at that time of year. A friend of mine decided that every year on her mother's birthday and death date, she and her family will go out to the movies—her mom's favorite activity.

VACATION TEMPTATION

In some small resort towns, summer tourists are often referred to as "fudgies" because when they're visiting, they feel they just have to buy fudge. Vacation time comes and we feel we just have go for the fudge, the ice cream (Double *scoop? Oh, what the hell, sure!*), and penny candy (*Ooo, they have those? I loved those when I was a kid! I'll take a pound of them! What? Twelve bucks?*). Like holidays, vacations are times to relax and be with people you love and care about, and break the old routine. Come up with some better ways to bond than consuming the junk food sold in every tourist shop. Bond over healthful meals. Enjoy cooking together or eating out at restaurants that have healthy food. Now you have access to menus and reviews on the Internet—you don't have to get stuck in the places that fry up foods and douse them in fatty sauces and serve them with bread made from processed flours. Ask for condiments on the side or bring your own.

I found some common issues discussed among my students around vacations and taking breaks in general. People who feel too much oftentimes don't know how to relax or take a break, owing to the familiarity of hypervigilance, always being on intuitive "patrol," and they can suffer from stability boredom when things become quiet. Being aware of this, if this is your tendency, it is important to be mindful of putting something in your mouth. Once you recognize the "poised for detour" behaviors, you can prevent yourself from sabotaging your progress.

TRIPPING UP WHEN ON A TRIP

I travel a lot for my work, and I've come to accept that the best way to eat healthfully is to bring, or purchase, snacks that are healthy and make them into meals. Again, you should try to figure out what restaurants near where you're staying serve healthy foods, but also, you might look up where the nearest grocery store is so you can pick up cheese (preferably organic and cruelty-free), nut butter, baby carrots, salads, celery sticks, fruit, and maybe some whole-grain or gluten-free crackers. I always travel with raw nuts and with packaged nutrition bars: I avoid the ones with textured vegetable protein (which is highly processed) and high carbs.

In most airports, the food kiosks between security and the gate have some fruits, yogurt, and salads, and sometimes they'll have hummus, too. If I don't have any cut vegetables to dip in the hummus, I'll use pretzels, which aren't a great choice but are okay in a pinch. It can be tricky to work around the rules for bringing liquids with you, but with a little planning, you can figure out how to have some good salad dressings or condiments available to you. Remember to bring a little bag or shaker of Himalayan salt everywhere you go.

Also, I always call the hotel I'm staying at and get them to clear the mini bar in my room, even if I have to pay for it. It's not worth the temptation to binge. After I've taken in the emotions and energy of a crowd of people, I like to retreat to my hotel room without those candy bars and bags of salty chips crying, "I'm here! Yummy yummy yummy! Let me comfort you! C'mon, no one will know!" Ask if there's a room without a mini bar. Find out if the nearby restaurants can serve you brown rice and steamed or grilled vegetables. Do the best you can and don't expect it to be perfect. Mindfulness, praying, and giving thanks for the food you are about to eat are powerful and good for your mind, body, and soul, regardless of whether you know where everything comes from. Freedom from obsession is the key, so don't sweat it if you can't access the perfect foods when you're on the go.

If you're overtired, which is very likely if you're traveling across time zones or you've had to spend an entire day or two getting to your destination, you'll be more susceptible to disordered eating. Figure out how you can take the time to ground yourself once you arrive, and shed all the emotional and energetic detritus that's clinging to you. I find it's easy to take a daily Himalayan salt bath whenever I travel, and it makes a huge difference in my ability to handle the stress of being on the road. If you can't access a tub, try to take a shower and use a salt scrub, or at least spritz and do the affirmations and your tapping. You might meditate a bit, too. Try not to schedule back-to-back meetings if you can. Even if you can just work in 10- or 15-minute breaks to be alone, away from anyone else's energy and your phone, the television, or other stimulation, you'll have an easier time managing your porous boundaries.

DEADLINES THAT OVERSTIMULATE YOU

For some people, an approaching deadline turns up the volume on their excitement, energy, and creativity. They do their best work in the wee hours before the project is due. I'm like that—an adrenaline junkie! I love having to go, go, go; but I also know that the high level of stimulation I feel when I've got a deadline hovering above me can lead me to feel ungrounded, which sets me up for disordered eating.

Now, other people completely shut down with anxiety as a deadline comes near, so they're better off getting started on the project right away and holding themselves to a strict schedule. Whatever your natural response to deadlines, the important thing is to know yourself and not to let any fear or frustration build up and cause you to go into emotional overload. If perfectionism is a problem, or your last-minute work usually needs a lot of tweaking, set yourself a false deadline ahead of the real one.

Then you'll have a cushion of time to play around with regarding your finished product, whether it's a book, a paper, or a presentation. Understand and accept the truth about how you work best instead of denying it.

Don't harshly judge yourself if you're bad with deadlines. As always, start with self-compassion. Then, your fear of failure won't interfere with your plan for how to get the work done on time. Procrastination stems from fear. Call it out into the open and work with it—as you sit in your salt bath, using the EFT, affirm, "Even though I am not a perfect writer (or speaker, or presenter), I deeply love and honor myself." In fact, use this technique before you sit down to write or get up to practice your presentation. I know that's going to be a little tricky when you're waiting to walk up to the podium, but you can dash into the bathroom to do it, and repeat the affirmations as you're sitting waiting to be called to the front of the room. Remember, there are only two main emotions, two sources of consciousness: fear that comes from the wounded ego and love, which is the natural state of your soul. The first is false, the other is true. Love is the answer to every question, and compassion is the attitude we should hold at all times—compassion for other beings and for ourselves. Love yourself even if your inner thoughts are churning with fear because you're afraid you won't make a deadline.

It's important to have deadlines in order to get done the larger or more difficult projects we would otherwise avoid. Our challenge is to decouple the deadlines from the emotional agitation we create around them. If the deadline was set by someone else, the fear of disappointing that person can be intimidating. If we set it and told someone about it, time seems to shrink because we fear we can't get the work done by that date. Because we're people pleasers, we also tend to overpromise. One habit a good friend of mine had to break was telling every client, "I'll get back to you tomorrow." It was an instant reaction to every request and it put enormous pressure on her. She learned that even if she thought she could get the task done in 24 hours, she could say, "I'll try to get back to you by the end of the week," and no one ever complained. Then, if she got back to the person the next day, or even the day after that, she looked good and felt good about herself. Do you have a habit of letting unrealistic promises pop out of your mouth automatically when you're anxious about pleasing someone else? Give yourself a time cushion and your emotions about deadlines will be quieter.

Also, if you're working with others on the project, be careful not to take on their agitation. You might be better off not partnering with someone who has a different response to deadlines than you do—early starters drive late starters crazy, and vice versa. If you're ready to go full steam ahead and your partner is looking at the amount of time you have left to complete your work and freaking out, it's not pretty. If *you* are the one who is anxious about time, try the Slowing Down Time exercise in Chapter 5 for relieving your anxiety and helping you to feel you have enough time to do what you need to do.

MAKING DECISIONS

Maybe your deadline involves making a decision. Weighing your options takes time, not just because you have to think through the pros and cons of your choice but also because you have to quiet the noise in your head and get in touch with your feelings about the decision. Are you upset that you have to make the decision in the first place? Change can be hard. If you can't get out of making a decision, and you don't like your options, soften your resistance and open yourself up to accepting that the circumstances have changed. After you make this internal shift, who knows? Maybe a new choice will present itself to you.

People who feel too much often have trouble with decisions because they pick up on everyone's feelings and don't want anyone to be hurt, upset, or angry so they procrastinate. *Maybe if I just think this through long enough, and poll enough people, I can find a solution that everyone will be okay with and we can all live happily ever after.* Let's face it, most people resist change, so the likelihood that you can reason your way into the perfect decision that no one disagrees with is approximately, oh . . . *next to nothing.* Let go of the illusion that you can please everyone and spend more time getting in touch with what your emotions are. Don't forget that you can always use the IN-Vizion Process and discover what the landscape that represents your feelings can teach you.

And be aware, too, that if you're very sensitive, you are likely to avoid the discomfort of acknowledging that something is wrong with the picture. If you stay on top of your emotions and manage your empathy, you can acknowledge problems early on in a situation and deal with them before the situation becomes completely unworkable and you're left angry, frustrated, and disappointed, with the decision taken out of your hands.

WHEN YOU ARE ILL

When you're not managing your porous boundaries very well, you're more likely to be stressed out, and as you learned in the section on adrenal glands, your body responds to stress by lowering your immune response. This can create a vicious cycle: you're feeling upset, anxious, irritated, or depressed; you get sick; then you're upset, anxious, irritated, or depressed because you're sick.

Being sick stinks, and emotional drama just makes me want to eat! Feed a cold, feed a fever—I want to feed it all to comfort myself!

Eating well and getting enough sleep boost your immunity and will bring you back to health more quickly, but worrying about how long it will be before you get better and indulging in comfort foods are just going to make matters worse. Do the Slowing Down Time exercise (see Chapter 5) if you feel yourself getting anxious, and use affirmations such as, "Even though I am achy, tired, and coughing, I still deeply love and accept myself" when taking your salt baths. Stay hydrated: drink plenty of liquids to help your body wash out the germs and toxins. Take this time to be good to yourself and to get in touch with any "emotional toxins" you are holding on to that could be contributing to your illness or fatigue. Do the Cord Unplugging exercise in Chapter 6 to see whether you are holding on to any emotions or energy that belongs to someone else, and cut the cords.

Don't pressure yourself to do a lot of exercise when you're sick. Get outside and walk if the weather is nice, but go for a shorter time and don't feel you have to get a workout. It's more important to keep the fluids in your body moving, stretch your muscles a bit, and use gentle exercise to manage your moods than to get your heart pumping. Don't weigh yourself because you might start to obsess about how you aren't burning calories. Think of this time as a temporary respite from all the stressors in your life, and as an opportunity to nurture yourself body, mind, and spirit. Okay, you can watch a little junk TV too, but rest and take care of your body and emotions.

LIFE CHANGES AND HORMONAL SHIFTS

For women, the hormonal shifts that happen during their menstrual cycle, in adolescence, and during perimenopause can make it especially difficult to manage emotions and empathy. A woman who has never experienced the mood shifts of PMS may be in for a shock when her estrogen levels drop in her late 40s, or after surgery that sends her into early menopause. But it's not just women who experience hormonal shifts that affect their moods. Men's sex hormones are at high levels in adolescence, then drop in midlife. They can experience irritability and depression during these shifts just as women can, but it's harder for them to talk about.

Men get the message loud and clear: be strong at all times, and don't show emotions because that's "weak." In fact, depression in men often manifests as anger, which feels like a powerful emotion because it makes people tiptoe around them when they express that anger; but of course, being angry all the time and not being able to control your rage is not powerful at all. A grouchy man in his 40s, 50s, and 60s who is overeating and gaining weight might be dealing with a hormonal shift, among other things (from feeling sad about growing older in a youth-oriented culture to regretting the mistakes of his youth that led to his current situation).

If you're in one of these stages of life when hormones shifts and life changes are normal, and you're noticing that you're more moody, sensitive, or angry, or less emotionally resilient, talk to your doctor about having your hormones tested. Hormone levels can be influenced by medications, but also by food, food supplements, exercise or movement, and other natural means. Don't underestimate the potential emotional stress that comes when your body and your life are changing at the same time that your hormone levels are shifting.

Then, too, women's hormone levels change dramatically in the hours and days after childbirth, which is why some women suffer from postpartum depression. It's also one of the reasons some women not only hold on to the baby weight but also have a much harder time losing weight than in the past. Becoming a parent is a huge life change, too. It's very easy for a woman to start neglecting herself so as to take care of the baby, to become emotionally overwhelmed by the challenge, and to detour into disordered eating, which doesn't exactly help with losing the weight. If you recently gave birth and are trying to lose weight, work the People Who Feel Too Much program, but check your hormones as well. Thyroid problems, which affect metabolism, often show up during these times of hormonal shifts, so I'll say it again: check your hormone levels, as it's likely they have changed and you're having new symptoms and more difficulty managing your emotions and your weight.

In adolescence, we detach from parents to form new, individual identities outside of the family. If you're very empathetic, this separation process is difficult because you are so intertwined with the emotions of your parents and siblings, but also those of your peers. Your best friend from childhood suddenly is interested in the opposite sex, not the games you two played together, and the rejection is excruciating. If you're empathetic, you're not only feeling your grief at the loss of a friendship, and maybe some embarrassment at being "immature" in her eyes, you're also taking on her discomfort with you and her resentment that you want her to go back to who she was last year.

When I was a young teenager, I had a very strong sense of being off-kilter. People told me I was oversensitive. In response, I decided to show everyone how tough I was, so I became rebellious. Then I had to deal with my burgeoning sexuality and with boys being attracted to me, which totally freaked me out. My desire for emotional intimacy was overwhelming, and I detoured away from it.

At the same time, I was developing bulimia. The effects of the manic binge would be erased by the conscientious purge—or at least, that's how it felt. It was frightening and exhilarating to engage in this secret behavior. The message I received was clear: fashionable, desirable girls were thin. I must have stepped on the scale twenty times a day, terrified that the needle might budge—and it did. No matter how much I threw up, I still gained weight and my curves still developed.

After I gained 20 pounds in one year, with no increase in height, I started on my first diet, which as I recall featured a lot of grapefruit. Then I went on a new diet every month, losing and gaining weight like a yo-yo. I hated my body and the pressure to control it was too much for me to bear. Drinking became a form of self-medication, and I started to identify with the wild, crazy, party girl persona I had created to disguise my deep discomfort with myself and my connections with other people and my body.

Teenagers who feel too much may not detour away from their feelings by using alcohol and drugs and acting out sexually, but they may start abusing themselves—cutting, embedding, and so on. These behaviors create a sense of being able to control intense feelings. Teens can also become very controlling and anxious. If their parents and the people around them give them good support and guidance, it can help them navigate these dangerous waters. If not, addictions may take hold and unhealthy detours can become coping mechanisms that then cause problems throughout adulthood. Did any of your addictions or detours start in your teen years? Are they affecting your son or daughter?

Many adults experience a midlife hormonal shift right when their kids are going through their own hormonal changes at adolescence. Just recognizing this and being willing to laugh about the challenge will help, but be aware of how using this program, and being on top of your hormone levels, can help you to help your kids manage puberty better. You might do some exercising together, or have media-free, stimulation-free times in the household, which will benefit everyone. Pay attention to what everyone's eating, and cook together so no one's tempted to escape to the fast-food joint for an emotional respite and some salty, fatty treats. Encourage your teens to use the techniques you're learning for managing porous boundaries. The daughter of one of my clients started doing Himalayan salt baths, and she found that they helped her shed the emotional crap she picked up each day in junior high school, and helped clear up her skin as well.

In ancient times, stories about the transition from maiden to mother to crone, or warrior (young man) to father to sage, helped people understand just how profound our life changes are and how challenging they can be. If you have a spiritual or religious tradition that marks these transitions, that's wonderful. Work with them! If you don't, you might want to create some rituals around them to help you, and the people you love, to experience just how big these shifts are and to honor them. Even if a woman or man doesn't become a literal mother or father, we enter into a stage where our bodies are fertile and we are expected to be mature role models for others, which we might not be emotionally prepared for, given where we are in our personal growth. Instead of retreating into denial and sensing shame about how we don't feel prepared to step into a new stage of life, we can find ways to honor it and ourselves, and make the change more easily.

Also in midlife, we often end up caring for elderly parents or family members, which can lead to adrenal burnout, as you learned about earlier. If you're in the sandwich generation, helping out your aging mom and dad while raising kids, maybe even teenagers, while you're in midlife—you've got quite a full plate! Be good to yourself.

CHANGES IN THE ELECTROMAGNETIC FIELD, AND LIGHT DEPRIVATION

As I mentioned earlier, we are all connected energetically to the energy fields around us, including the electromagnetic field (EMF) of the earth. If you're very sensitive, you might be picking up on the many changes within the larger electromagnetic field and experiencing changes in your emotions. It wasn't so long ago in human history that no one had electric lighting, much less computers and electronic devices, radio waves, and technologies that affect the EMF. Now, you can't go anywhere without someone using an electronic device near you. Our bodies and our energy fields have had little time to adjust to the alterations to the energy fields that surround us.

Using the salt baths, and keeping salt water and salt lamps in areas where you have electronic equipment, will help balance the electromagnetic field by releasing negative ions (remember: negative ions good, positive ions bad). But it's also important to reduce the amount of energy disturbance you expose yourself to. I know that I am much more emotionally sensitive and empathetic when I feel overwhelmed by the "buzz" in the electromagnetic field created by all of our technologies. This happens frequently when I'm in cities or crowded spaces. If you have to be around a lot of electronic equipment, make sure to take breaks and to use your techniques for managing your porous boundaries. I'm not saying that the crowd of people at the airport using their cell phones and computers are making you fat, but they are affecting you energetically—even more than they would in a previous generation, when people in public spaces had to communicate with the office by dropping a coin into a pay phone.

If you think about it, we lead very unnatural lives, and we may be grossly underestimating how much our energy fields are being affected. For example, we have exposure to light all hours of the day, but it's often not natural lighting. The spectrum of a fluorescent or even an incandescent lightbulb is limited, so the light is very different from sunlight.

If you live in a part of the world where the natural light is low much of the year—for example, if you're very far north or south of the equator—you aren't getting much vitamin D from sunlight. The same is true if you rarely get out into natural sunlight, or only do so during certain times of the year. Low levels of vitamin D are associated with depression and a host of physical problems, from fatigue to cognitive impairment to diabetes and cancer. Also, when we spend more time in sunlight, particularly on bright sunny days, we have higher levels of serotonin, a "feel-good" neurotransmitter that our brain needs to regulate mood.

The solution is to get out into the sunshine, and if you are especially sensitive to low levels of natural light, consider buying a light box and natural-spectrum lights to use in your home or office. Seasonal affective disorder (SAD) is a very real phenomenon that affects people who do not get exposed to enough natural light, influencing their moods; it seems to be very common among people who feel too much. If you get more depressed and lethargic on dull winter days, or during the rainy season in your area, learn more about SAD and get some sun! It will help you to avoid unnecessary sadness that can cause you to detour away from healthy eating and emotional management.

NATURE DEPRIVATION

Just five minutes spent in nature can improve a person's mood, according to research; and there's growing evidence that exercising in nature instead of indoors provides extra benefits for mood. If you're like many people, you spend a lot of time inside. Do you find you only know what the weather is if you go to your iCal or check a website, because you're too far away from a door to step outside and find out for yourself how cold, sunny, rainy, or windy it is? We've become so detached from nature!

Getting outside and into nature is important. If you hate the cold or you have trouble handling it because of an underlying condition, bundle up with lots of layers of clothing and forget about how unfashionable you look. If you can't stand getting wet or feeling the wind against your bare skin, find clothing that works for you. If you're afraid you'll ruin your hairstyle in the wind or rain, find a way around it so you can get the sunlight and the time around trees, sky, creeks, dirt, and animals that your spirit, mind, and body need. Check into whether there are indoor gardens in your area that you could visit, too. Why not take a few spins around the botanical gardens or enjoy the miniature desert under the skylights? Maybe there's a public aquarium nearby where you can spend some time sitting on a bench, watching the fish and the seahorses. It can really make a difference in your mood and sense of calm. Many of the participants in my workshops for People Who Feel Too Much have reported that getting in touch with nature regularly is incredibly effective for managing their porous boundaries. So, don't let the weather stand in your way. Bring nature indoors, too, with plants, fountains, pets, and windows to the outdoors.

MOON CYCLES

During certain moon cycles, emotions run higher than at other times. In fact, *lunacy* comes from the Latin root *luna,* or "relating to the moon," because it was believed that a full moon made people a little crazy. Although research has disproved the urban myth that there are more ER visits and nervous breakdowns during a full moon, an especially sensitive person might be affected by the moon's phases. After all, women's menstrual cycles are somehow connected to and perhaps influenced by moon cycles.

I can always feel a full moon coming, as if it were singing through every cell in my body, and more often than not, I have an increase in mood swings around the full moon. New moons make me feel like starting new things. You might find the same is true for you. There are many online resources for lunar calendars, and you might want to pay attention to the moon's cycles and see if they correlate to your moods. If they do, you can be prepared for needing a little extra self-nurturing when the moon enters a phase that seems to make you irritable or sad. As always, be mindful of what affects you emotionally, and be self-compassionate when it comes to your sensitivities.

Over the years, I have come to be more and more open-minded and to view my experiences with curiosity, looking for consistency in the repetition. I don't believe everything I am told, but if I experience something to be true, even if I don't fully understand the "how" of it, I rely on the evidence. We people who feel too much have experiences that allow us to trace the invisible threads that for so long have made us question our place in the tapestry of life, wondering if we're cuckoo when reaching for the cookie jar, anxious for relief. As we come to listen more to our own inner wisdom, it will be easier for us to shut out the external noise, including the harsh judgments and unreasonable demands others may make of us. Instead of anticipating others' disappointment and twisting ourselves into knots trying to please everyone before they can experience irritation or anger that we know we'll pick up on, we can relax in knowing that we have control over our porous boundaries. We have the tools to clearly demarcate where we end and where others begin.

I hope that this book has helped you claim your true sense of power and granted you a healthier sense of connection to the world. I especially hope you've now solved the puzzle of your empathy, your habit of taking on the cares of the world and struggling with your weight. Just remember to be compassionate and kind to yourself and others. Your fabulous self is right inside you!

KEEP IN MIND . . .

- There will be especially challenging times when it's particularly difficult to manage your porous boundaries and avoid disordered eating.
- Remember that celebrations don't have to be about food as entertainment.
- Cut gatherings short or take breaks from them. Introduce new, healthier foods to celebrations that involve eating. Come up with new traditions for celebrating that don't involve eating noisy foods. At family gatherings, steer conversations away from hot topics, and keep your sense of humor.
- Be prepared for strong emotions and feelings of vulnerability to come up on anniversaries of losses and around the holidays.
- When you're on holiday, don't take a vacation from eating healthfully.
- Plan for healthy snacks and meals when you know you're going to be traveling.
- Recognize the emotional pressures that deadlines create and the tendency for that adrenaline rush to drive you into disordered eating. Be aware that people who are working with you, who handle deadlines differently from how you do, can cause you stress, too, and manage your porous boundaries.
- When feeling pressed by time, use the Slowing Down Time exercise (Chapter 5).

- When you have to make big decisions, recognize that you can't please everyone. Watch that you don't procrastinate in order to avoid making a decision that someone might not agree with.
- When you're sick, get some movement to prevent aches and pains, and don't let yourself start worrying about getting work done or whether you're gaining weight.
- Work with medical professionals, nutritionists, and the like if you suspect your hormones are off because of going into or being in menopause, having given birth, or being a man in midlife. Know that teenagers also go through hormonal shifts that affect their moods, weight, and ability to manage their emotions well without detouring.
- Changes in the electromagnetic field that surrounds you can affect you. Use Himalayan salt lamps to balance the ionization in the electromagnetic field.
- Natural-light deprivation can affect your moods and energy. Use full-spectrum lightbulbs and lamps to address seasonal affective disorder (SAD) and mood problems caused by low light levels. Make sure you're getting enough vitamin D, which the body creates when exposed to sunlight.
- Not spending time outdoors, being nature deprived, can affect your mood. Spending just five minutes in nature can boost it.
- Some people who feel too much are strongly affected by moon cycles.

Whatever the challenge to manage your porous boundaries, continue to use the basics of this program:

- setting your intention in the morning and, in the evening, reflecting on your day and something positive that you did, and journaling whenever you feel a need to speak your truth
- getting regular movement
- being kind to yourself, using the IN-Vizion Process, and any other exercises you find helpful (such as Slowing Down Time)

- doing the Emotional Freedom Technique as an alternate technique any time you have an extra minute or two
- incorporating Himalayan salts into your daily life, especially through a salt bath, and making sure your emotional field and eating remain simple

Afterword:
Moving Forward
to a Fabulous You

As you take your place in this wonderful dance called life, you'll come to recognize that you are indeed "one" with everyone else on this earth. After working this program, you'll feel less and less driven by the need to shut down and detour away from the exquisite, intense connection that empathy brings. Freedom is something you can feel deeply, from the depths of your soul, as you come to recognize that only love is real and that the fear that kept you a prisoner in your wounded self was an illusion.

As people who feel too much, we can take our place in the global community, recognizing that our empathy is something that is beginning to take shape in everyone as we evolve into a civilization more interconnected and more collaborative than at any other time in human history. We are a sentient species that has now populated the whole world. Will empathy bring peace and a better way of life? I hope so.

What I have learned is what you will learn, too. Life is never perfect, and it's a day at a time that you need to concern yourself with, not a lifetime. As you take care of yourself each day, you are helping to foster a new, healthier experience for everyone on this planet. Deal with the weight you can carry, not with the weight of the world.

I have come to understand that there is a huge paradox we collectively experience: the wounded ego somehow bought into the illusion that we are separate, not whole—and unsafe. When we feel too much, we have a sense of urgency to disconnect from ourselves, from each other, and from Spirit. Yet more separation is not the answer. A boundary isn't a wall; it's a structure created by our conscious decision to trust ourselves and experience our self-worth. It supports our individual expression, which is central to our human experience. We are meant to feel and to express the true reality of our nature, which is unity and Love.

We can have healthy boundaries that are fluid and flexible while we experience the world with deep and profound sensitivity, and we don't have to end up with our face in the fridge, trying to escape. Love is the only true reality; when we know this, everything changes.

Going forward, there are three things you need to remember. First, forgiveness isn't something you do when you feel like it. It's mandatory. You can't walk around in your life holding resentments and expect to feel freedom at any level. Let go of your emotions about the past that are no longer helping you and only weighing you down. Hold on to the wisdom you have achieved as a result of your suffering, and the compassion you have for others who have suffered, too.

If you refuse to forgive, you will continue to be fat. Release the emotional weight of a past you can't change. Otherwise, your fear will be your companion and it will rob you of peace and self-respect. All human beings suffer and hurt each other when they buy into the illusion that there isn't enough, that intimacy is unsafe, and that retaliation and anger are the only ways to protect the treasures of the heart.

Second, faith is not just something for church. You are the church. Your faith in a power greater than yourself is an action, not an idea, because faith is surrender. You surrender your life to that higher power, God, Spirit, or whatever name you have for the force you believe in that is beyond your comprehension, and peace, miracles, and magic follow. Every day, you can be awed by the mystery. Remember, you are part of that and there is a plan for you. Act as if you believe in magic, and it will come to pass that you will see the signs everywhere. I know this to be 1000 percent true, as it has happened to me.

Third, be grateful. You are living in exceptional times. Now is the time for you to claim your fabulous self and show her or him to the world. Shake that tail! Dance as if you mean it and laugh every day! Don't take yourself so seriously, and above all don't let others dictate to you what size you should be or what kind of beautiful you need to be to be accepted. Who makes those ridiculous rules anyway? If you can see the humor in the absurdity of it all, you'll be free to be your wonderful, fabulous self. You will hold the key to expressing the divine spark inside you that has been waiting to come out, maybe for your whole life.

I bet you're awesome.

Notes

CHAPTER 1: FEELING TOO MUCH: THE HIDDEN THREAD

15 *You probably see other people in shades of gray rather than black or white, and you don't overidentify with one separate group.* Ernest Hartmann, *Boundaries: A New Way to Look at the World* (Summerland, CA: CIRCC EverPress, 2011), p. 5.

16 *African-American women are three times as likely . . . to be overweight.* Mark Penn, with E. Kinney Zalesne, *Microtrends: The Small Forces Behind Tomorrow's Big Changes* (New York: Twelve, 2007), pp. 181–83: "According to a 2002 study in the *Journal of the American Medical Association* (JAMA), women in general are about twice as likely as men to be morbidly obese, but a sobering 1 in 6 black women is that overweight—almost more than three times the prevalence rate for any other subgroup of women or men. . . . According to a 2006 JAMA study, morbidly obese people tend to be concentrated in the 50 to 59 age group, which means the heaviest black women are in their working and grandmothering prime. And here's the worst part. Also according to the JAMA study, which tracked its subjects for seven years, middle-aged, morbidly obese women had almost double the chance of dying during the study than women of normal weight. That puts middle-aged black

women at perhaps one of the highest mortality risks in the nation." Penn goes on to say, "Although black women make up only about 6 percent of the U.S. work force, they make up 7 percent of all educational service workers. They make up 23 percent of America's service industry overall. Black grandmothers are raising or helping to raise 44 percent of the black children in America—well above twice the grandmother raising rate of any other racial group in America."

26 *Aron . . . estimates the number of highly sensitive people to be around 20 percent. . . .* Elaine Aron, *The Highly Sensitive Person: How to Thrive When the World Overwhelms You* (New York: Broadway Books, 1997), pp. 28–29. In citing the 20 percent figure, Aron references her own research, as well as that of Harvard psychologist Jerome Kagan.

26 *. . . 845 million . . . people are on Facebook.* 845 million people out of 7 billion is about one in eight, or 12 percent. See https://www.facebook.com/press/info.php?statistics (retrieved March 27, 2012).

CHAPTER 2: WHEN YOU CARRY THE WEIGHT OF THE WORLD

30 *Studies by the HeartMath Institute . . . show that our brain waves respond to electromagnetic signals from the heart of a person in the same room with us.* Rollin McCraty, Ph.D., "The Energetic Heart: Bioelectromagnetic Communication Within and Between People," in *Clinical Applications of Bioelectromagnetic Medicine,* edited by P. J. Rosch and M. S. Markov (New York: Marcel Dekker, 2004), pp. 541–62; http://www.heartmath.org/research/research-publications/energetic-heart-bioelectromagnetic-communication-within-and-between-people.html.

33 *you can actually get your heart to entrain to the rhythm of music just by listening to it.* Don Campbell and Alex Doman, *Healing at the Speed of Sound: How What We Hear Transforms Our Brains and Our Lives* (New York: Hudson Street Press, 2011).

33 *"The world essentially operates . . . in the connection between [things]."* Lynne McTaggart, *The Bond: Connecting Through the Space Between Us* (New York: Free Press, 2011), p. xxv.

34 *had one member of a couple send loving, healing thoughts to the other. . . . [W]hen two people were in separate rooms with their eyes closed. . . .* Ibid. McTaggart cites her lengthier description of these two

experiments in Chapter 4 of her previous book, *The Intention Experiment: Using Your Thoughts to Change Your Life and the World* (New York: Free Press, 2007), pp. 56–61.

34 *For people who feel too much, emotions and thoughts are always intertwined.* Ernest Hartmann, *Boundaries: A New Way to Look at the World* (Summerland, CA: CIRCC EverPress, 2011), p. 47.

35 *the leaf began to emit biophotons.* . . . This is just one of many "intention" experiments writer Lynne McTaggart has conducted along with scientists. See Lynne McTaggart, *The Intention Experiment: Using Your Thoughts to Change Your Life and the World* (New York: Free Press, 2007). See also: http://www.theintentionexperiment.com/wp-content /uploads/2011/01/The-Leaf-Experiment.pdf.

39 . . . *seventeen years for research to make its way into mainstream clinical practice.* J. A. Mold and K. A. Peterson, "Primary Care Practice-based Research Networks: Working at the Interface Between Research and Quality Improvement," *Annual of Family Medicine* 3, Supplement 1 (May–June 2005): S12–20. See also: http://www.childrens mercy.org/stats/weblog2005/SeventeenYears.aspx (retrieved March 7, 2012).

CHAPTER 3: THE WEIGHT LOSS FOR PEOPLE WHO FEEL TOO MUCH PROGRAM

45 *Showing kindness toward yourself, having self-compassion, is more effective than willpower when it comes to sticking to your eating goals.* Claire E. Adams and Mark R. Leary, "Promoting Self-Compassionate Attitudes Toward Eating Among Restrictive and Guilty Eaters," *Journal of Social and Clinical Psychology* 26, no. 10 (2007): 1120–44; http:// guilfordjournals.com/doi/abs/10.1521/jscp.2007.26.10.1120.

45 . . . *willpower can be depleted quickly; exercising willpower uses glucose (sugar).* Kelly McGonigal, Ph.D., "The Science of Willpower," *IDEA Fitness Journal* 5, no. 6, (June 2008); http://www.ideafit.com /fitness-library/science-willpower-0.

45 *social stress makes it harder to exercise willpower.* . . . *getting enough quality sleep and being in a good mood boost willpower, as does eating well and getting movement.* Ibid.

47 *The tapping slows the heart rate.* . . . Much research has been done

on EFT and how it works, and we're continuing to learn more about how this combination of tapping meridian points, acknowledging our problems, and affirming that we love ourselves is so effective. See Dawson Church, Ph.D., Garrett Yount, Ph.D., and Audrey Brooks, Ph.D., "The Effect of Emotional Freedom Technique (EFT) on Stress Biochemistry: A Randomized Controlled Trial," *Journal of Nervous and Mental Disease*, in press. See also David Feinstein, Ph.D., "Rapid Treatment of PTSD: Why Psychological Exposure with Acupoint Tapping May Be Effective," *Psychotherapy: Theory, Research, Practice, Training* 47, no. 3 (2010): 385–402; James Lane, Ph.D., "The Neurochemistry of Counter Conditioning: Acupressure Desensitization in Psychotherapy," *Energy Psychology: Theory, Research & Treatment* 1, no. 1 (2009): 31–44. These and other research articles on EFT, including three that show EFT helps alleviate food cravings, are available through http://www.eftuniverse .com/index.php?option=com_content&view=article&id=18&Item id=21 (accessed May 15, 2012).

49   *. . . regularly acknowledging what you're grateful for will make you happier, healthier, and more optimistic.* John Tierney, "A Serving of Gratitude May Save the Day," *New York Times*, November 21, 2011; http://www.nytimes.com/2011/11/22/science/a-serving-of-gratitude -brings-healthy-dividends.html?_r=1.

53   *Keep in mind that whatever you experience in these places in your mind, you're always in charge.* In my book *The Map*, I wrote about using the IN-Vizion Process to explore landscapes and dialogue with archetypal beings that dwell within them, such as the Goblin and the Bone Collector. Even when you encounter a being in your inner landscape, it is only an aspect of yourself and you are always in control of the experience. Colette Baron-Reid, *The Map: Finding the Magic and Meaning in the Story of Your Life* (Carlsbad, CA: Hay House, 2011).

56   *Negative ions are believed to affect serotonin levels in our brains.* M. C. Diamond, J. R. Konner Jr., E. K. Orenberg, et al., "Environmental Influences on Serotonin and Cyclic Nucleotides in Rat Cerebral Cortex," *Science* 210, no. 4470 (November 7, 1980): 652–54; http://www .sciencemag.org/content/210/4470/652.abstract.

56   *. . . research suggests that people who have thin boundaries . . . are especially sensitive to changes in the ionization in the environment.* Michael Jawer, "Environmental Sensitivity: A Neurobiological Phenomenon?" *Seminars in Integrative Medicine* 3, no. 3 (September 2005):104–9.

Jawer, an expert on indoor air quality and workspace management, says there's a connection between positive ion buildup and migraines, fatigue, irritability, anxiety, and depression, and says that people who report to be "electrically sensitive" often report sensory sensitivities and mystical and paranormal experiences.

58   *[Four o'clock] is when our blood pressure naturally peaks.* Robert B. Sothern, D. L. Veseley, E. L. Kanibrocki, et al., "Blood Pressure and Atrial Natieuretic Peptides Correlate Throughout the Day," *American Heart Journal* 129, no. 5 (May 1995): 907–16; http://www.ahjonline.com /article/0002–8703(95)90111–6/abstract). See also, L. E. Sheving and F. Halberg, *Chronobiology: Principles and Applications to Shifts in Schedules* (Norwell, MA: Kluwer Academic, 1981). Blood pressure, body temperature, and heart rate are highest "in the afternoon," according to J. C. Dunlap and Jennifer J. Loros, *Chronobiology: Biological Timekeeping* (Sunderland, MA: Sinauer Associates, 2009), pp. 341–45.

61   *Just spending five minutes walking or exercising outdoors can improve your mood.* Jo Barton and Jules Pretty, "What Is the Best Dose of Nature and Green Exercise for Improving Mental Health? A Multi-Study Analysis," *Environmental Science & Technology* (2010): 100325142930094, DOI: 10.1021/es903183r (retrieved from: http://www.sciencedaily.com/releases /2010/05/100502080414.htm). Also http://pubs.acs.org/doi/abs/10.1021 /es903183r (retrieved March 25, 2012).

65   *. . . bottles of soda pop or servings of salty snacks that are 50 to 60 percent larger than they were thirty years ago.* Between 1977 and 1998, soda pop serving sizes went up 50 percent and salty snacks went up 60 percent. S. J. Nielsen and Barry M. Popkin, Ph.D., "Patterns and Trends in Food Portion Sizes: 1977–1998," *Journal of the American Medical Association* 289, no. 4 (2003): 450–53.

65   *. . . women who watch three to four hours of television a day. . . .* L. A. Tucker and M. Bagwell, "TV Watching and Obesity in Adult Females," *American Journal of Public Health* 81, no. 7 (1991): 908–11. Compared to women who watched on average one hour of television a day, women watching three to four hours a day were twice as likely to be obese, and women watching four or more hours a day were more than twice as likely to be obese.

67   *. . . unsuspecting subjects who ate from a soup bowl. . . .* Brian Wansink, J. E. Painter, and J. North, "Bottomless Bowls: Why Visual Cues of Portion Size May Influence Intake," *Obesity Research* 13 (2005):

93–100 (retrieved from: http://www.nature.com/oby/journal/v13/n1/full
/oby200512a.html).

CHAPTER 4: STEP ONE: SPEAK YOUR TRUTH

110   *Cinematherapy.* Counselors often use cinematherapy as a way to help
their clients experience their emotions at a distance, as they watch them
played out in someone else's story on-screen, then talk about what that
experience was like. You can also watch movies to remind yourself that
your life isn't so bad after all and to connect with a feeling of gratitude.
S. Knobloch-Westerwick, Y. Gong, et al., "Tragedy Viewers Count Their
Blessings: Feeling Low on Fiction Leads to Feeling High on Life," *Communication Research*, March 26, 2012. Cinematherapy was popularized
by the humorous series of books of the same name written by Peske and
West; see Nancy K. Peske and Beverly West, *Cinematherapy: The Girl's
Guide to Movies for Every Mood* (New York: Dell, 1999).

112   *. . . many people who feel too much also experience physical sensations more intensely. . . .* Elaine Aron, *The Highly Sensitive Person:
How to Thrive When the World Overwhelms You* (New York: Carol Publishing Group, 1996), p. 7.

113   *U.S. Navy SEALs . . . replac[e] negative self-talk with positive
affirmations.* http://information.usnavyseals.com/2009/07/learning-to
-learn-the-navy-seals-way.html (retrieved March 23, 2012).

113   *In moments of stress, there's actually more blood flow to [the limbic
brain].* See David Perlmutter, M.D., F.A.C.N., and Alberto Villoldo,
Ph.D., *Power Up Your Brain: The Neuroscience of Enlightenment* (Carlsbad, CA: Hay House, 2011).

CHAPTER 5: STEP TWO: OWN YOUR TRUTH

123   *These flavorings seem to train the palate. . . .* For an eye-opening
and an unsettling portrait of just how much chemical tinkering goes
into fast food, see Erich Schlosser, *Fast Food Nation: The Dark Side of the
All-American Meal* (New York: Houghton Mifflin, 2001), pp. 121–31.

133   *Meditation . . . helps with depression and anxiety.* http://www
.psychologytoday.com/articles/200304/the-benefits-meditation   (retrieved March 24, 2012).

133　*research led by Sara Lazar, Ph.D., showed that mindfulness meditation . . . thickening the regions [in the brain] associated with. . . .* This landmark study was conducted on people who had never meditated before. Changes were found in the posterior cingulate cortex (where self-awareness and empathy are experienced), the left hippocampus (involved in memory), the cerebellum (involved in language, focus, and motor control), and the temporal-parietal junction. See "Mindfulness Practices Lead to Increases in Regional Brain Grey Matter Density."

134　*The temporal-parietal junction [may be] the part [of the brain] where we experience a sense of ourselves. . . .* Andrew B. Newberg, Ph.D., *Principles of Neurotheology* (Burlington, VT: Ashgate Publishing, 2010), p. 175.

135　*"A man's eyes cannot be as much occupied as they are in large cities by artificial things. . . . "* Quoted in Charles E. Beveridge and Paul Rocheleau, *Frederic Law Olmsted: Designing the American Landscape*, edited and designed by David Larkin (New York: Rizzoli, 1995), p. 34.

CHAPTER 6: STEP THREE: RECLAIM YOUR POWER TO CHOOSE

166　*[Laughter] relieves tension and stress.* Mayo Clinic Staff, "Stress Release from Laughter? Yes, No Joke," http://www.mayoclinic.com/health/stress-relief/SR00034 (retrieved March 25, 2012).

167　*[Laughter] opens your blood vessels.* Michael Miller and William F. Fry, "The Effect of Mirthful Laughter on the Human Cardiovascular System," *Medical Hypotheses* 73, no. 5 (November 2009): 636–39.

167　*[Laughter] possibly preventing heart attacks.* University of Maryland Medical Center, "Laughter Is the Best Medicine for Your Heart," http://www.umm.edu/features/laughter.htm (retrieved March 25, 2012).

CHAPTER 7: STEP FOUR: RECONNECT WITHOUT LOSING YOURSELF

181　*"Muscle burns fat. . . . "* Julia Ross, M.A., *The Diet Cure* (New York: Penguin Books, 2000), p. 217.

184 . . . *movement prevents . . . panic attacks.* A. J. Smits, Candyce D. Tart, et al., "The Interplay Between Physical Activity and Anxiety Sensitivity in Fearful Responding to Carbon Dioxide Challenges," *Psychosomatic Medicine* 73, no. 6 (July 2011): 433; http://www.psychosomatic medicine.org/content/73/6/498.short. See also: http://www.sciencedaily .com/releases/2011/07/110712122403.htm (retrieved March 25, 2012).

184 *According to a theory called* sensory integration. . . . See Lindsey Biel, OTR/L, and Nancy Peske, *Raising a Sensory Smart Child: The Definitive Handbook for Helping Your Child with Sensory Processing Issues* (New York: Penguin Books, 2009): 12–18. Although it's a book for parents who want to help their kids, it is full of information that applies to adults with sensory issues, including ideas for accommodations and heavy work activities that adults would enjoy.

186 . . . *whole-body vibration . . . boost[s] circulation, immunity, and the flow of your bodily fluids.* . . . My husband, Marc, and I are so impressed by the research on the effects of whole-body vibration that we've invested in Goga Studios, which features whole-body vibration machines. See the Goga Studios research page on their site: http://www .gogastudios.com/technologyResearch.html; see also: http://www.ncbi .nlm.nih.gov/pubmed/15472009.

187 *According to the Centers for Disease Control, walking at a good clip.* . . . The Centers for Disease Control and Prevention, "How Much Physical Activity Do Adults Need?" http://www.cdc.gov/physicalactivity /everyone/guidelines/adults.html (retrieved March 25, 2012).

188 *Movement has an even greater effect on our spirits and attitude when we exercise outdoors.* J. Thompson Coon, K. Boddy, et al., "Does Participating in Physical Activity in Outdoor Natural Environments Have a Greater Effect on Physical and Mental Well-being than Physical Activity Indoors? A Systematic Review," *Environmental Science Technology* 45, no. 5 (February 3, 2011): 1761–72; http://pubs.acs.org/doi/abs/10.1021 /es102947t (retrieved March 25, 2012).

188 . . . *being in nature offers a host of health benefits.* Jules Pretty, Ph.D., "How Nature Contributes to Mental and Physical Health," *Spirituality and Health International* 5, no. 2 (June 2004): 68–78; http://onlinelibrary .wiley.com/doi/10.1002/shi.220/abstract (retrieved March 25, 2012).

189 . . . *having too many fat cells lowers your metabolism while increased muscle mass raises it.* The Mayo Clinic Staff, "Metabolism and Weight Loss: How You Burn Calories," http://www.mayoclinic.com/health/ metabolism/WT00006 (retrieved March 25, 2012).

190   *Perimenopausal and menopausal women, and people who have ex-
       perienced excessive emotional or physical stress.* . . . Marcelle Pick,
       M.D., *Are You Tired and Wired?: A Proven 30-Day Program for Over-
       coming Adrenal Fatigue and Feeling Fantastic Again* (Carlsbad, CA: Hay
       House, 2011).

191   *. . . sleep deprivation lowers your metabolism and makes it harder
       to lose weight.* Kelly McGonigal, Ph.D., "The Science of Willpower:
       In Defense of a Good Night's Sleep," *Psychology Today,* October 29,
       2009; http://www.psychologytoday.com/blog/%5Bfield_blog_ref-title
       -raw%5D/200910/in-defense-good-nights-sleep (retrieved March 25,
       2012).

192   *. . . 70 to 90 percent of people with certain common autoimmune
       disorders are female.* In her book *Women's Bodies, Women's Wisdom,*
       Dr. Christiane Northrup points out that 70 percent of multiple scle-
       rosis sufferers are female, 75 percent of rheumatoid arthritis suffers are
       female, and 90 percent of lupus erythematosus are female. Christiane
       Northrup, M.D., *Women's Bodies, Women's Wisdom: Creating Physical
       and Emotional Health and Healing* (New York: Bantam Books, 2010),
       p. 816. The National Institutes of Health's website says that women make
       up 70 percent of autoimmune hepatitis sufferers. See: http://digestive
       .niddk.nih.gov/ddiseases/pubs/autoimmunehep/ (retrieved March 25,
       2012).

192   *. . . the prolonged stress of caretaking can lead to autoimmune disor-
       ders.* See: http://www.nccdp.org/article-planning-for-eldercare.htm.

194   *. . . every time you do something habitual, like get into your car to
       start it, or stand at the sink to brush your teeth.* . . . Peggy McColl,
       *Your Destiny Switch: Master Your Key Emotions, and Attract the Life of
       Your Dreams!* (Carlsbad, CA: Hay House, 2007), pp. 166–67.

196   *Subscribe to "good news only" news services.* See http://www.goodnews
       network.org and http://www.happynews.com.

CHAPTER 8: NOW LET'S TALK ABOUT FOOD

212   *[Livestock] are also given antibiotics.* . . . The concern about the
       excess use of antibiotics has grown so great that the Obama admini-
       stration is pressuring American farmers to stop using them. Gardi-
       ner Harris, "Steps Set for Livestock Antibiotic Ban," *New York Times,*
       March 23, 2012; http://www.nytimes.com/2012/03/24/health/fda-is

-ordered-to-restrict-use-of-antibiotics-in-livestock.html?_r=1&scp
=1&sq=antibiotics%20livestock&st=cse.

213   *. . . people would rather deny that an animal they eat has suffered
than change their eating habits.* Steve Loughnan and Brock Bastian,
"The Role of Meat Consumption in the Denial of Moral Status and
Mind to Meat Animals," *Appetite* 55, no. 1 (2010): 156.

215   *. . . most North Americans eat more protein than they need.* The
Centers for Disease Control and Prevention, "Nutrition for Everyone:
Protein";   http://www.cdc.gov/nutrition/everyone/basics/protein.html
(retrieved March 25, 2012).

218   *. . . scientists in Britain and France have recently discovered that
a common pesticide is killing off much of the bee population. . . .*
Carl Zimmer, "Two Studies Point to Common Pesticide as a Culprit in
Declining Bee Colonies," *New York Times*, March 29, 2012. http://www
.nytimes.com/2012/03/30/science/neocotinoid-pesticides-play-a-role-in
-bees-decline-2-studies-find.html?scp=1&sq=bee%20pesticide&st=cse.

218   *Is it a coincidence that American girls are entering puberty before
age 10. . . .* Elizabeth Weil, "Puberty Before Age 10: A New 'Normal'?" *New York Times*, March 30, 2012; http://www.nytimes.com/2012
/04/01/magazine/puberty-before-age-10-a-new-normal.html?scp
=1&sq=female%20puberty&st=cse.

221   *List of foods that are lowest and highest in pesticides.* The Environmental Working Group, "EWG's 2011 Shopper's Guide to Pesticides in
Produce." http://www.ewg.org/foodnews/summary/ (retrieved March 25,
2012).

223   *Many spices not only bring flavor to your food but are also incredibly
healthy for you.* Ni Shing and L. Ac Mao, D.O.M., Ph.D., "5 Spices
to Invigorate Energy and Health." http://www.doctoroz.com/blog/mao
-shing-ni-lac-dom-phd/5-spices-invigorate-energy-and-health (retrieved
May 14, 2012). Also, Mike Adams and Dani Veracity, "Natural Appetite
Suppressants for Safe, Effective Weight Loss," eBook (Truth Publishing, 2009); http://www.naturalnews.com/downloads/NaturalAppetite
Suppressants.pdf. Also, Joseph Mercola, M.D., "Top 10 Anti-Aging Herbs
and Spices," http://www.doctoroz.com/videos/top-10-anti-aging-herbs
-and-spices (retrieved May 14, 2012).

225   *. . . fructose (too much) and fiber (not enough) appear to be cornerstones of the obesity epidemic. . . .* UCSF Mini Medical School for the
Public, *Health and Medicine*, July 2009, Show ID 16717.

232 *Some food cravings have a physical component.* See, for example, Philip Werdell, M.A., "Physical Craving and Food Addiction: A Scientific Review," *The Food Addiction Institute,* 2009; http://foodaddiction institute.org/scientific-research/physical-craving-and-food-addiction-a -scientific-review/ (retrieved May 14, 2012).

CHAPTER 9: CHALLENGING TIMES FOR PEOPLE WHO FEEL TOO MUCH

248 *Cheap, processed food can be found around the globe now, even in India. . . .* Karishma Vyas, "Expanding India Faces Obesity Problem," *ChinaDaily.com.cn,* March 19, 2011; http://www.chinadaily.com.cn /cndy/2011–04/19/content_12350128.htm.

268 *women's menstrual cycles are somehow connected to and perhaps influenced by moon cycles.* E. Friedman, "Menstrual and Lunar Cycles," *American Journal of Obstetrics and Gynecology* 140, no. 3 (June 1, 1981): 350. http://www.ncbi.nlm.nih.gov/pubmed/7246643. See also: Sung Ping Law, "The Regulation of Menstrual Cycle and Its Relationship to the Moon," *Acta Obstetricia et Gynecolegia Scandinavica* 65, no. 1 (1986): 45–48; http://informahealthcare.com/doi/abs/10.3109 /00016348609158228.

Recommended Reading
and Resources

DOCUMENTARIES

Food, Inc.: How Industrial Food Is Making Us Sicker, Fatter, and Poorer—And What You Can Do About It. Dir. Robert Kenner. Magnolia Home Entertainment, 2009. DVD.

Food Matters. Dir. James Colquhoun and Carlo Ledesma. Passion River Films, 2009. DVD.

Forks Over Knives. Dir. Lee Fulkerson. Virgil Films and Entertainment, 2011. DVD.

Fresh. Dir. Ana Joanes. New Video Group, 2012. DVD.

The Tapping Solution. Dir. Nicolas Ortner. The Tapping Solution, LLC, 2009. DVD.

FIND A WEIGHT RELEASE ENERGETIX COACH

I am very proud to announce that on my website www.micicoach.com, as well on my personal site, www.colettebaronreid.com/weightloss, you will be able to find a friendly, supportive, compassionate, well-trained coach to personally guide you through this program! My certified Weight Release Energetix coaches are trained to specifically help people who feel too much to manage their emotions, providing unique and cutting-edge methods to remove the blocks to their greatest success while entering into a weight-loss program. Coaches gently guide you through a deeper and more thorough experience with the IN-Vizion Process as they help you create the space for your transformation. You will find a list of coaches, their websites, and their contact information, as well as details about their other skills so you can choose who you feel is the best fit for your needs.

IN-VIZION PROCESS FOR WEIGHT LOSS DOWNLOADS

Can't afford a coach and like to do things on your own? There are many recorded versions of the IN-Vizion Process to help with weight release and empathy overload, available on my site for download.

Listening to these sessions daily may greatly improve your success!

And we have awesome support tools to help you at home and on the go! Kick-start your success with one of our Weight Release Transformation Project's most popular classes available for download:

"Your New Best Friend—The Hidden Secrets to Weight Release Revealed!"
Visit www.colettebaronreid.com/weightloss.

BOOKS

Aron, Elaine. *The Highly Sensitive Person: How to Thrive When the World Overwhelms You.* New York: Carol Publishing Group, 1996.

Baron-Reid, Colette. *The Map: Finding the Magic and Meaning in the Story of Your Life.* Carlsbad, CA: Hay House, 2011.

Biel, Lindsey, OTR/L, and Nancy Peske. *Raising a Sensory Smart Child: The Definitive Handbook for Helping Your Child with Sensory Processing Issues.* 2nd. ed. New York: Penguin Books, 2009.

Blaylock, Russell, M.D. *Excitotoxins: The Taste That Kills.* Santa Fe, N.M: Health Press, 1997

Braden, Gregg. *Secrets of the Lost Mode of Prayer: The Hidden Power of Beauty, Blessings, Wisdom, and Hurt.* Carlsbad, CA: Hay House, 2006.

———. *The Spontaneous Healing of Belief: Shattering the Paradigm of False Limits.* Carlsbad, CA: Hay House, 2008.

Campbell, Don, and Alex Doman. *Healing at the Speed of Sound: How What We Hear Transforms Our Brains and Our Lives.* New York: Hudson Street Press, 2011.

Craig, Gary. *EFT for Weight Loss: The Revolutionary Technique for Conquering*

Emotional Overeating, Cravings, Bingeing, Eating Disorders, and Self-Sabotage. Fulton, CA: Energy Psychology Press, 2010.

Dossey, Larry, Ph.D. *Space, Time & Medicine.* Boston: Shambhala Books, 1982.

Freedman, Rory, and Kim Barnouin. *Skinny Bitch.* Philadelphia, PA: Running Press, 2005.

Hartmann, Ernest. *Boundaries: A New Way to Look at the World.* Summerland, CA: CIRCC EverPress, 2011.

Karr, Chris. *Crazy, Sexy Diet: Eat Your Veggies, Ignite Your Spark, and Live Like You Mean It.* Guilford, CT: skirt!, 2011.

Linn, Denise, and Meadow Lynn. *The Mystic Cookbook: The Secret Alchemy of Food.* Carlsbad, CA: Hay House, 2012.

Lipton, Bruce, Ph.D. *The Biology of Belief: Unleashing the Power of Consciousness, Matter, & Miracles.* Carlsbad, CA: Hay House, 2011.

Masson, Jeffrey Moussaieff. *The Face on Your Plate: The Truth About Food.* New York: W. W. Norton & Co., 2009.

———. *The Pig Who Sang to the Moon: The Emotional World of Farm Animals.* New York: Ballantine Books, 2004.

McColl, Peggy. *Your Destiny Switch: Master Your Key Emotions, and Attract the Life of Your Dreams!* Carlsbad, CA: Hay House, 2007.

McTaggart, Lynne. *The Bond: Connecting Through the Space Between Us.* New York: Free Press, 2011.

———. *The Intention Experiment: Using Your Thoughts to Change Your Life and the World.* New York: Free Press, 2007.

Newberg, Andrew B., Ph.D. *Principles of Neurotheology.* Burlington, VT: Ashgate Publishing, 2010.

Northrup, Christiane, M.D. *The Wisdom of Menopause: Creating Physical and Emotional Health During the Change.* Rev. ed. New York: Bantam Books, 2012.

———. *Women's Bodies, Women's Wisdom: Creating Physical and Emotional Health and Healing.* New York: Bantam Books, 2010.

Orloff, Judith, M.D. *Emotional Freedom: Liberate Yourself from Negative Emotions and Transform Your Life.* New York: Three Rivers Press, 2010.

———. *Positive Energy: 10 Extraordinary Prescriptions for Transforming Fatigue, Stress, and Fear into Vibrance, Strength, and Love.* New York: Three Rivers Press, 2005.

Perlmutter, David, M.D., F.A.C.N., and Alberto Villoldo, Ph.D. *Power Up Your Brain: The Neuroscience of Enlightenment.* Carlsbad, CA: Hay House, 2011.

Pert, Candace. *Molecules of Emotion: The Science Behind Mind-Body Medicine.* New York: Simon and Schuster, 1999.

Peske, Nancy K., and Beverly West. *Cinematherapy: The Girl's Guide to Movies for Every Mood.* New York: Dell, 1999.

Pick, Marcelle, M.D. *Are You Tired and Wired?: A Proven 30-Day Program for Overcoming Adrenal Fatigue and Feeling Fantastic Again.* Carlsbad, CA: Hay House, 2011.

Ross, Julia, M.A. *The Diet Cure: The 8-Step Program to Rebalance Your Body Chemistry and End Food Cravings, Weight Gain, and Mood Swings—Naturally.* New York: Penguin Books, 2012.

———. *The Mood Cure: The 4-Step Program to Take Charge of Your Emotions—Today.* New York: Penguin Books, 2003.

Schlosser, Erich. *Fast Food Nation: The Dark Side of the All-American Meal.* New York: Houghton Mifflin, 2001.

WEBSITES

Services that offer only good news include the
Good News Network http://www.goodnewsnetwork.org
and Happy News http://www.happynews.com.

You can also find good news on the *Huffington Post* at
http://www.huffington post.com/good-news/.

You can find a list of farmers' markets in your area at this site:
http://apps.ams.usda.gov/FarmersMarkets/.

Here is the website of Feng Shui master Angel de Para:
http://www.earthluck.org.

SELF-HELP GROUPS

Alanon Family services
http://www.al-anon.alateen.org
Codependents Anonymous
http://www.coda.org
Overeaters Anonymous
http://www.oa.org

For information on nutrition, check the following websites:
http://www.cdc.gov/nutrition/everyone/index.html
http://www.droz.com
http://www.drweil.com
http://www.mercola.com
http://www.metagenics.com

Acknowledgments

This book has many to thank for its birth.

To my genuine, creative, hilarious, always-faithful husband, Marc Linde-man, you will always have my forever love.

I offer my . . .

Deep abiding gratitude to Jennifer Rudolf Walsh for truly being my fairy godmother, believing in me, showing me I could be more in the world, bringing me to Crown, but most important for becoming the best kind of friend—honest, steadfast, and true. I love you so much.

Great thanks to my fabulous agent Andy McNichol. You are a smart, savvy, wondrous being and really great agent! I adore you.

Giant and most major thanks to Tina Constable, Julia Pastore, and every-one at Crown Archetype publishers, whose support and wonderful enthusiasm for my work were palpable when I walked in the door. Thank you for all your support and hard work to make this book fly.

My admiration and great gratitude to Nancy Peske, my developmental edi-tor extraordinaire. This is our third project together, and it keeps getting better all the time.

A big, giant hug and major thanks to my team at the Master Intuitive Coach Institute: Michelle Morgan, Kim Johnson, Mark Johnson, Jay Appleby.

A giant HOORAY to all the certified Weight Release Energetix coaches and students who are helping others who feel too much recognize that there is a way out of the empathy overload and a way back into a decent size pair of pants!

To all my dear friends, thanx for your support as I struggled to write this while surrendering that the cookie jar will not help with my anxiety about how this book will be received. I love you all so so much. You know who you are. ;)

Index

About the Author

Colette Baron-Reid is an internationally respected intuitive counselor, coach, and life strategist with a client base spanning twenty-nine countries. She is the author of numerous bestselling transformational wellness and mind/body spirit products, audio programs, and books including *The Map: Finding the Magic and Meaning in the Story of Your Life*. She has been a popular featured guest on radio and TV, appearing on *Dr. Phil*, Oprah and Friends with Dr. Mehmet Oz and Lisa Oz, *Coast to Coast AM*, and others. She is the host of two popular weekly call-in radio shows on the CBS-owned New Sky Radio.

She lives happily and gratefully between the U.S. and Canada with her husband and two tiny fur-covered children dressed up in Pomeranian suits. Visit her at her website, www.colettebaronreid.com.

0000121800312